DR. CAPUTI'S PRINCIPLES FOR NURSE EDUCATORS

ALSO BY DR. CAPUTI

Think Like a Nurse:
The Caputi Method for Learning Clinical Judgment
(USA Version)

Think Like a Nurse:
The Caputi Method for Learning Clinical Judgment
(Canadian Version)

Certified Nurse Educator Review Book:
The Official NLN® Guide to the CNE Exam
(2nd Edition)

DR. CAPUTI'S PRINCIPLES FOR NURSE EDUCATORS

A GUIDE FOR TEACHING NURSING

Dr. Linda Caputi

Dr. Caputi's Principles for Nurse Educators:
A Guide for Teaching Nursing

Windy City Publishers
www.windycitypublishers.com

Printed in the United States of America

ISBN:
978-1-953294-39-5

Library of Congress Control Number:
2023902545

Cover Image by udra11/Shutterstock.com

WINDY CITY PUBLISHERS
CHICAGO

This book is dedicated to all nursing faculty and nursing students everywhere.

For over four decades, I have dedicated my work life to nursing students and nursing faculty.

I could not have chosen a better place to work.

Dr. Linda Caputi, MSN, EdD, CNE, ANEF

DR. CAPUTI IS PROFESSOR EMERITUS, College of DuPage in Illinois. She has taught in LPN, ADN, BSN, and MSN programs. She is President of Linda Caputi, Inc., a nursing education consulting company. Across nearly three decades, Dr. Caputi has consulted with over a thousand nursing schools on topics related to teaching clinical judgment, revising curriculum, developing a new curriculum, transforming clinical education, test item writing and analysis, student retention, increasing NCLEX pass rates, and numerous other nursing education topics. She has also presented at over 1,000 workshops and nursing education conferences. Dr. Caputi has won six awards for teaching excellence from Sigma Theta Tau, is included in 3 years of *Who's Who Among America's Teachers*, was nominated for the Outstanding Teacher Award in 2005 from the National League for Nursing (NLN), and was presented the 2004 Educator of the Year Award from the Organization of Associate Degree Nursing.

For ten years Dr. Caputi served as the editor of the Innovation Center, a column in the NLN's journal *Nursing Education Perspectives* and has served on the NLN's Board of Governors. Dr. Caputi is a Certified Nurse Educator and was inducted as a fellow into NLN's Academy of Nursing Education.

Throughout her career, Dr. Caputi has published numerous books, book chapters, journal articles, educational software programs, online learning materials, and even board games for nursing students. She is the editor of the 2nd edition (2020) of the *Certified Nurse Educator Review Book: The Official NLN Guide to the CNE® Exam* and 5 other books published by the National League for Nursing. She co-authored with Dr. Jean Giddens, *Mastering Concept-based Teaching* (1st and 2nd editions). The 2nd edition of her three-volume book *Teaching Nursing: The Art and Science* won the 2010 Top Teaching Tools Award in the print category from the *Journal of Nursing Education*.

Dr. Caputi is the author of *Think Like a Nurse: The Caputi Method for Learning Clinical Judgment* (2022), a textbook for nursing students. This text actually teaches what clinical judgment is and presents a very detailed framework for students to use when applying clinical judgment to nursing content to plan individualized, quality patient care and for preparing for the clinical judgment aspect of the Next Generation NCLEX. This text is used in all levels of Registered Nursing Programs and Practical/Vocational Nursing programs. Dr. Caputi also authored the Caputi Online Clinical Judgment Course for use by nursing programs that adopted the textbook to ensure all students are consistently learning clinical judgment. To learn more visit: https://LindaCaputi.com.

Dr. Caputi, assisted by Lesley MacMaster, authored the Canadian version of *Think Like a Nurse: The Caputi Method for Learning Clinical Judgment.* Professor McMaster adapted the entire text to ensure it aligns with standards of nursing practice in Canada. This text is used in Canadian Registered Nursing and Practical Nursing programs. To learn more visit https://lindacaputi.com/about-the-book/ and scroll down to the "Canadian Version" section of the page.

Dr. Caputi's website https://LindaCaputi.com includes a blog and more information about all the services and products Dr. Caputi has available.

CONTENTS

NCLEX, NCLEX-RN, and NCLEX-PN are registered trademarks
of the National Council of State Boards of Nursing (NCSBN).

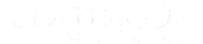

INTRODUCTION

THE PURPOSE OF THIS BOOK is to offer some basic or fundamental principles for all nurse educators. In this book, I consider a principle to be the guiding basis for conduct in one's practice. For me, these principles represent the rules or methods to use when engaged in the many and varied roles of a nurse educator.

One of the major themes throughout this book is for faculty to consider why they are doing what they are doing. Faculty often "teach as they were taught" without questioning or understanding the true implications for what is being done. One of the Principles in the chapter "Teaching and Learning Practices" is "Always know the WHY behind the WHAT." My hope is this book will take some of the unknown out of what we do as nurse educators and look to the question, "Why do we do that?" This is one of the pleasures I experienced working with new faculty. Many would often ask that question. That question forced me to reflect: "Yeah, exactly why am I doing that?" We must know the educational "why" we are doing something as a beginning piece of evidence for what we are doing.

> Always know the WHY
> behind the WHAT.

I developed the principles in this book based on lessons learned in the MSN and EdD programs which I completed; my own teaching practices; consultations with schools of nursing across 49 states, Washington, DC, and Canada; and immersion in nursing education literature. The first book I wrote of this nature was titled *Little Lessons for Nurse Educators*. This current book translates some of those lessons into basic principles which can be used to guide actions and behaviors as a nurse educator.

Little Lessons for Nurse Educators was light-hearted and, hopefully, inspirational. *Dr. Caputi's Principles for Nurse Educators* takes on a more serious tone. Much has changed in nursing education over the 16 years since the initial book was published. Much has changed in nursing practice. There are new educational theories such as Retrieval Theory that can greatly benefit nursing education. New educational tools are available. Nurse educators demonstrated great strength, endurance, and resiliency when the pandemic required faculty to swiftly transform from face-to-face to online delivery across all learning environments. Nurse educators showed they can change when change is needed.

On the other hand, nurse educators can be resistant to change. Outdated or ineffective practices related to clinical education, standardized testing, classroom teaching/learning strategies, and many other practices continue to be used even though there is no research to support many of those practices. Because there are many new ways of doing, all those involved in nursing education must be open to new ideas and be willing to let go of the known and implement change when change is needed. A fair, accurate, and honest assessment of collected data is required to identify the need for change—then change must be implemented to maintain quality nursing programs.

To meet the goal of considering new ways of doing, this book presents detailed principles related to the topics covered in each chapter. These principles can be used and even tweaked as needed by administrators and faculty teaching at all levels of nursing education. Although much of the book is focused on specifics related to pre-licensure nursing programs, the principles are applicable to all nursing education programs. For example, when talking about teaching to prepare students for the NCLEX, the same principles can be applied by faculty teaching in graduate nursing programs preparing students for a certification exam written upon graduation.

It is time for all in nursing education to reflect on our past practices, determine what works and what does not work, then select, create, and implement new ways of doing to move our practice, our students, and nursing education forward. Remember, before an idea is considered a "brilliant idea," it often was considered a "crazy" idea.

My professional pleasure is to watch as the current generation of nurse educators is redefined. These nurse educators will no longer be those who say, "But this is the way it has always been done," but rather, "Let's reimagine, rethink, rebuild, and renew nursing education by using new ways of doing—new ways to make our nursing education world a better place to be." I believe this is a very achievable goal. For some readers I hope to plant seeds that will grow into new and better ways of doing. For other readers, I hope to plant the idea that perhaps the way we have always engaged in nursing education can be changed to make nursing education even better than what we are currently providing.

Let's reimagine, rethink, rebuild, and renew nursing education by using new ways of doing— new ways to make our nursing education world a better place to be.

Who You Are as a Nurse Educator

ALL NURSE EDUCATORS KNOW WHO they are as a nurse. They have a well-defined self-concept of themselves as a professional nurse. This is important because it provides the basis for performing in a nursing position. Your self-concept guides your actions based on the values and roles you use to define yourself as a nurse.

Faculty new to education must define who they are as a nurse educator. What are your values and roles? What do you do as a faculty member? What guides your practice?

Most experienced faculty have a well-defined self-concept of themselves as faculty. However, the role of the nurse educator changes as nursing, students, and education changes. Adapting to change means growing as a nurse educator which influences your self-concept as an educator. Your self-concept as a nurse educator will change over time as you adapt and adjust to new ways of doing.

The Principles in Chapter 1 speak to the roles, values, and behaviors of a nurse educator. For some readers these may be new ideas; for others, they may reinforce your already established self-concept as a nurse educator. May the Caputi Principles help you self-reflect and reconsider who you are as an educator. In whatever way you use them, I hope you find them helpful as you grow in your role as a nurse educator.

Chapter 1 Principles

The Principles in this chapter will help you define who you are as a nurse educator, and adapt to the ever-evolving nursing environment.

PRINCIPLE

#1 Enjoy the moment; enjoy your moments of success in your role as a nurse educator.

Have you ever heard the saying, "If you need music on the beach, you're missing the point. The enjoyment is in what you are doing?"

In 2022 at his televised 100th birthday party Norman Lear (creator of hit TV shows such as *All in the Family*) was asked to share some advice about life. He answered to "always appreciate the moment." The past is over, the future is next, but it is in this middle time of the here and now where you are actually present. Always take the time to enjoy the moment.

We are always so busy in our teaching that we sometimes do not enjoy the moments with our students. The happy moments in teaching must be captured and remembered. The memory of those moments helps you through the tougher times. Those moments are your rewards as a teacher. It is a joy to witness someone transforming from a new student entering the nursing program to new nurse entering the profession. That trans-

> The happy moments in teaching must be captured and remembered.

formation is one of the highlights, the joy, a moment of pure pleasure for a nurse educator—and knowing you may have had a little something to do with that transformation.

PRINCIPLE

#2   Use the language of a student-centered teacher.

As with all interactions, the type of language faculty use with students contributes to students' success. Positive language reflects the culture of the nursing program and communicates who you are as a nursing faculty. For example, faculty should use language such as:

- "How can I help?" Asking students how you can help shows you are sincere about their learning and you are willing to share your time with them.

- "What do you think?" Asking students what they think demonstrates an interest in them and gives them a chance to share what they know. This fosters confidence.

- "Your success is my priority. Let's talk about what you can do to improve your grade." Individualized help shows you care about the person. Faculty-mediated help shows you care about the student.

Helping students succeed involves faculty providing support and guiding students through remediation activities. The trend in nursing education has shifted from faculty providing "remediation" (filling in gaps of knowledge and thinking abilities) to faculty assigning third-party vendor products such as those from a standardized testing company or resources that accompany a textbook. Non-faculty review may or may not provide what students need. Students need an individualized plan about what to study and review to fill in any knowledge gaps. Delegating student remediation to a third-party vendor may not convey to students a sincere faculty concern for their success.

> Show in both your words and your actions your sincere concern for students.

5

In the Appendices of this book is the *Loma Linda Exam Analysis Tool**. Using that tool students identify lots of factors that interfered with earning a passing score on an exam. In the research conducted by Condon, et al (2016), one of the factors that students commonly identified was the need for better faculty support. The faculty support these authors recommend consists of psychological support such as caring, understanding, encouraging growth, being approachable, and demonstrating empathy. Faculty behaviors that reflect psychological support include being available to talk with students, engaging in clear communication, providing helpful feedback, using fair evaluation methods, helping students identify problems and resolutions, and serving as role models. Faculty support can **significantly** affect student success. All these behaviors reflect a "student-centered" culture.

Show in both your words and your actions your sincere concern for students.

*More discussion about using the *Loma Linda Exam Analysis Tool*
is included throughout this book.

PRINCIPLE

#3 When we stop caring about our students, it's time to leave.

I've had a nagging orthopedic issue for several years. The physician has tried many different treatments but nothing is helping the discomfort. The purpose of a recent office visit was to discuss any remaining treatment options. When the physician entered the exam room, another person was with him. The physician introduced the other person as a physician just starting his residency in orthopedics. I'll call him Dr. So and So. As my physician interacted with me and examined me, I noticed that Dr. So and So was tapping his fingers on the counter, looking out the window, and occasionally looking over his left shoulder and gazing into a mirror. He was definitely not focused on me and not even listening to the conversation. I interrupted my physician and asked Dr. So and So to please leave the room. In surprise he pointed to his chest and asked, "Me?" I answered, "Yes, I think it best for you to leave."

When I left the office Dr. So and So was in the hall in front of me and we entered the elevator at the same time. We were the only two people on the elevator. He said to me, "I'm sorry if I offended you." He just opened the door—this is my chance to teach. I shared with him that I have been a nurse for over 40 years and have worked with many physicians—some of whom are caring and some of whom are not. I shared that his non-verbal behavior definitely put him in the latter group. I said to him, "You may not have learned this in medical school or were perhaps absent for the discussion, but let me just share an important lesson with you. Don't ever think you are better than the patient." He just nodded and quietly said, "Okay."

This healthcare provider was a physician, but this story is not about physicians, it is about all healthcare providers. My experience just happened to be with a physician. All healthcare providers must be caring and empathetic even if not particularly interested in the patient's situation. When the caring stops, it's time to leave.

This Principle applies to the faculty-student relationship. When we stop caring about our students, it's time to leave.

PRINCIPLE

#4 Ensure that students will always think of you as someone who made them feel good.

I've learned that people will forget what you said,
people will forget what you did,
but people will never forget how you made them feel.

~Maya Angelou

A student shared with me her story of earning a GED. When she was 16 years old, she became pregnant and dropped out of high school. Her family was very poor so she worked to support herself and her baby while at the same time earning her GED. When she walked across the stage to receive her GED, rather than receiving a "Congratulations," the person handing the document to her said, "I don't know why you bothered." The student was devastated. However, she shared that she told herself, "That person let me down, but I won't let it bring me down." She enrolled in the nursing program where I taught and shared that story with me. I was, of course, shocked. Of the thousands of students I have taught, she was one of the most motivated, brightest students I have had the pleasure of teaching. But she will never forget how that person made her feel.

> People will never forget how you made them feel.

PRINCIPLE

#5   Earning certification as a nurse educator is a mark of excellence.

In the first two decades of my teaching career, some professional nursing organizations did not recognize the academic nurse educator as an advanced practice specialty. The National League for Nursing has debunked that belief with the "advanced specialty role of the academic nurse educator" (Halstead, 2019, p. 3). The advanced specialty role of the academic nurse has similar expectations as other advanced practice roles. These include a broad knowledge base, core competencies, and a certification exam.

At the time of this writing, the National League for Nursing has three certification examinations available for nurse educators: Certified Nurse Educator, Certified Academic Clinical Nurse Educator, and Academic Novice Educator. All three certification exams designate a mark of quality and excellence. The National League for Nursing has designated the nurse educator as an advanced practice nurse (Adams, 2015). If nurse educators are considered advanced practice nurses, then certification should be a requirement for the role. My advice is to confirm your role as an advanced practice nurse and become certified.

> The academic nurse educator
> is an advanced practice nurse.

PRINCIPLE

#6
Be curious and grow from your inexperience.
Find an area of nursing education that interests
you and become an expert.

People often ask me how I became a nursing education consultant. My simple answer is that I was curious. I was always curious about the details of every aspect of nursing education and worked to learn as much as I could. The more I learned, the broader my perspective grew in any particular area. I looked outside of what was happening at the school where I taught. I sought to learn how educators at other schools around the country were involved in the same activities I was involved with. I faithfully read four nursing education journals.

I was curious about everything and worked to learn more. Curriculum development is an example. In the late 1990s I was asked to help a school revise their curriculum. I declined because I had never revised a curriculum and did not feel prepared. But I was curious about what curriculum revision meant and how to do it. I read everything I could find about curriculum revision, attended conference presentations, and talked with colleagues at other schools. I reviewed documents such as the state Nurse Practice Act rules and regulations for nursing programs

> Be curious about
> what you don't know;
> keep on the path of
> learning and growing
> as a nurse educator—
> you never know where
> that path might take you!

and nursing accreditation standards to learn what was required. I compared and contrasted curricula at all levels of nursing education and from various nursing programs.

In 2006 my dean asked me to write the curriculum for a new nursing program that would need state board of nursing approval prior to offering the program. The dean also stated the college wanted that new program to earn nursing accreditation with the first cohort graduating from the new program. I readily accepted the challenge because I could now use everything I had learned. I was able to enjoy the experience, feel confident in what I was doing, and create a new program.

The new program was approved on the first submission to the state board of nursing. ACEN visited in the last semester of the program of the first cohort, and the program achieved ACEN accreditation for the first graduating class. ACEN's final report indicted the program was fully compliant with all standards and criteria and there were no identified areas in need of improvement. Since that time, I have consulted with hundreds of nursing programs across the United States at all levels of nursing education.

Curiosity about what I did not know and had no experience with provided the motivation and the desire to learn and I was able to reap the rewards—even to this day. Be curious about what you don't know; keep on the path of learning and growing as a nurse educator—you never know where that path might take you!

PRINCIPLE
#7 Nurse educators are "real" nurses.

Throughout my decades long teaching career, I would be asked: "What do you do?" My answer would be that I teach nursing at the local college. The response often was, "Oh, that's nice. Are you a real nurse?"

Real nurses teach nursing! How could we possibly teach others to become nurses if we are not nurses? I'm not sure of the genesis of this error in thinking. We need to spread the word!

Not only are nurse educators "real" nurses, but we are also advanced practice nurses.

Real nurses teach nursing!

PRINCIPLE

#8 Keep your passion for nursing education alive; be flexible.

We must be flexible in life and in nursing education. In the late 1990s, I listened to a keynote delivered by Dr. Malone, the Chief Executive Officer of the National League for Nursing. I remember Dr. Malone saying, "Flexibility can fuel your passion for nursing education!"

At the time she delivered the keynote she was working in Washington, DC with the American Nurses Association. Her keynote topic was about the importance of being flexible. She shared the story of when she was to meet with President Clinton. The meeting was set for 1 PM. She felt it necessary to eat before meeting with the President so she would not get light-headed during the meeting. As she ate a bowl of soup, she spilled some on her suit. She was to meet with President Clinton in 15 minutes. She did not want to meet with soup on the front of her suit. What will she do? Here is what she said:

> Flexibility can fuel your passion for nursing education!

"Someone walked by my door. She looked about my size. I said to her very nicely, 'Can I see you for a minute? I need your clothes.' I have a lovely picture of me with President Clinton, and I was in someone else's clothes." What a great example of flexibility!

PRINCIPLE

#9   Teaching nursing is NOT a retirement job!

I have met many nursing faculty over the years who confided in me saying that leaving practice and taking a nursing faculty position was to be their "retirement job." A "retirement job" is perceived to be less hectic than a current practice position and eases the person into retirement. However, one faculty shared that after accepting the "retirement job" position, that she did not have a degree in nursing education, and quickly realized she had been unaware of the full scope of faculty responsibilities. She stated she thought her role as faculty would be to go in the classroom and talk about what was in the textbook augmented by her experience as a nurse, then write some test questions. She had no idea the degree of complexity of the nurse educator role. However, it did not take her long to realize that teaching nursing was not the "retirement job" she was expecting.

The academic nurse educator
role is very complex.

PRINCIPLE

#10 Growing by small steps can lead to success as a nurse educator.

So much of what we do as faculty, and so much of what students do, isn't really serving either party very well. Simple changes can make a big difference. All nursing faculty want to be successful and want their students to be successful, but very few faculty are aware there are little things they can do every day that can lead to success.

Of course, there are many big changes that can make a huge difference in the quality of a nursing program. Less than desirable program outcomes may indicate that big changes are needed. However, big changes are difficult to implement and take time. There are times when big changes need to be made, but as we are waiting for the changes to be complete, and the effects of those changes realized, faculty can make some smaller, simpler changes.

Some of the simple changes faculty can implement that can make a big difference are discussed in the book *Make it Stick* by Brown, Roediger, and McDaniel (2014). This book is full of simple changes that can greatly influence the success of students— both in terms of completion rates and NCLEX/Certification Exam pass rates.

> Simple changes can greatly influence the success of your students.

Make it Stick talks about teaching so students are able to recall previously learned information. Now wouldn't that be nice! A common complaint in nursing education is that students do not remember what they learned in earlier course work. This issue has been a point of discussion across all the decades I have been in nursing education and it still exists. Perhaps if this problem has existed for such a long time, it may have more to do with teaching/learning practices than students unable to recall previously learned information. *Make it Stick* teaches about retrieval theory. It provides insights and ideas for how to engage students in active retrieval of previously learned information. This was a big "Ah-ha" moment for me when I read this book.

Throughout this book I discuss various aspects of retrieval theory in the context of other Principles. Retrieval theory is very powerful and should be used consistently across nursing programs at all levels.

As you read through this book, you will learn many small steps you can take as you continue to develop as a nurse educator. Highlight the teaching/learning strategies that can be implemented fairly quickly. List those out. Talk with your faculty colleagues about them. Work collaboratively to make the changes.

The Workplace

NURSING EDUCATION RESIDES IN MANY types of workplaces. I have visited a vast number of schools over the decades of my consulting. The physical workplace of nursing education programs varies greatly. Some nursing programs are housed in buildings that range in age from brand new to over 100 years old. Some schools have amazing technology, elaborate furnishings, and gorgeous artwork. Other schools have minimal technology, bare walls, and sparce furnishings.

The facilities themselves do not make the workplace. Facilities must provide students what they need to learn and teachers what they need to teach. However, the nature of the physical needs and facilities depends on the program. All schools have what they need because they are approved by their state boards of nursing and/or education boards to operate and most are accredited by nursing accreditation organizations. The physical elements of the workplace are provided.

The element of the workplace this chapter addresses is not the physical facilities. The element of the workplace this chapter addresses is the **culture** of the workplace. The culture is what makes the workplace what it is; what gives the workplace its nature, personality, and desirability. The culture is established by people, maintained by people, and broken by people. A positive, harmonious workplace culture is most productive. A positive workplace culture supports not only faculty but also students. The intent of the Principles in this chapters is to support faculty as they grow in a positive, harmonious workplace.

Chapter 2 Principles

The Principles in this chapter help you establish a positive, harmonious workplace culture to support both faculty and student success.

PRINCIPLE

#1   The culture of the workplace matters.

Workplace culture refers to the overall mood, tone, or ambiance within a workplace. Civility (politeness, courtesy) can greatly impact workplace culture. Civility refers to interactions between faculty and students; students and faculty; faculty and faculty; and faculty and administrators. Civility flows both ways between two people or groups of people.

Many nursing education settings have experienced a variety of incivility issues. There is student to faculty incivility, faculty to student incivility, and even faculty to faculty incivility. Incivility in any form sets the stage for failure.

Students come in many types and varieties. Some students are quite reserved and polite. Others are less reserved and less polite. Students come from very different backgrounds and experiences. Students who are already licensed should have learned the lessons of civil conduct within a profession; however, we cannot expect all student to behave in the way we believe they should behave upon entering a pre-licensure nursing program. Faculty have the very important job of teaching all students professionalism and professionalism requires civility.

The culture of the work environment lays the foundation for how we interact with other faculty and how we interact with students. We must have a "can do," student-centered, colleague-supportive environment. This culture must be across all aspects of the nursing program—higher level administration, nursing program administration, faculty, and all nursing program staff. That culture should be guided by principles of civility.

Build a culture of civility for everyone in your nursing program. Ensure all are informed of the expected behaviors. Many schools include a civility policy in their Nursing Student Handbook. The policy typically lists the behaviors expected when students interact with each other and with faculty. However, what must also be included are the behaviors expected of faculty as they interact with students. Faculty must always conduct themselves in a civil manner and sometimes civility isn't so obvious or intuitive. For example, if you are meeting with a student in your office and the phone rings or your cell phone sends out the audio notification of an incoming text, will you pause even for a quick moment to look at who the call or text is from or will you ignore the call or the text notification and totally focus on the student? Even briefly turning your attention to the phone tells the student they are not as important as that incoming call or text. If you are waiting for a call or text that requires your immediate attention, inform the student of the situation at the onset of your meeting. Small behaviors can send strong messages.

> Include a Civility Policy
> in both your
> Nursing Student Handbook
> and your
> Nursing Faculty Handbook.

It is also important to include a civility policy in your Nursing Faculty Handbook. The civility policy provides information about how all involved in the nursing program are expected to treat each other. There are times when habits of our everyday lives infiltrate our interactions with others in the nursing program. These habits may be acceptable in everyday life but likely not acceptable in a professional environment. For example, what is the expected behavior during nursing faculty and nursing committee meetings? Should faculty be grading papers while others are speaking? What about reading and responding to text messages? I have served on several boards over the last decade and I was somewhat surprised when I witnessed board members texting during meetings. At one point the Chair of one of the boards declared board meetings as "no-texting" time. Not a bad idea.

PRINCIPLE

#2 After writing an angry email, read it carefully; then delete it.

There is enough discord, anger, and rudeness already in the world, why add to it? Most behaviors that arise from anger are not productive or helpful; they are a waste of time. There is no place in nursing education for anger. There are problems in nursing education—but none of which can be solved through anger. Every day when you are at work, you are creating your future work environment. What kind of place do you want your work environment to be? One filled with anger? One filled with collegiality? We make these decisions every day; let's create a good future work environment.

I was always amazed when I received angry emails from fellow nursing faculty. Email is a one-way communication. Perhaps the person writing the email does not realize the degree of anger expressed in their email, but the anger is there. And the anger and negativity are in writing in perpetuity, which actually puts the sender at risk for repercussions as a result of the angry email. One email I received was from a nursing faculty who was angry at students. She sent the email to all nursing faculty and even to the nursing administrator.

> Who wants to teach in a workplace culture built on anger and negative thoughts about students?
>
> What does that accomplish?

Her perception was students were not reading all the chapters assigned because they were not motivated, dedicated, or independent learners. She sent the email using the college email system, and stated that she is tired of this type of student. She then called the students, "The cream of the college crap." Shocking.

It is important to note that not once did that faculty look to herself to determine what she might do to improve the situation. If this situation is happening with many cohorts of students, the problem may not be a student problem. Perhaps it is the homework assignment itself that is not meaningful so students are not motivated to read 300 pages and "come to class prepared." What does "come to class prepared" even mean? The topic of meaningful homework assignments is discussed in Chapter 4.

Writing angry emails is a bad idea for the reasons presented: (1) an angry email does not accomplish anything positive, (2) an angry email puts the sender at risk for professional harm.

Never send an angry email and be careful what you put in writing.

PRINCIPLE
#3   Stay calm in the workplace.

Ducks are interesting. They appear calm on the water's surface yet they paddle like crazy underneath. As nurses, we have learned to be ducks as a patient's condition deteriorates. We give the appearance of calm, while our minds are speeding forward to collect all the data we'll need to determine what to do next.

This same situation happens in education. It will happen in your relationship with students. It will happen in your relationship with faculty colleagues. It will happen in your relationship with administrators. All these groups will say things or make decisions that might trigger an emotional response. We must remain calm on the surface. Remaining calm is a necessity for clear thinking. We must remain calm and think through problems to arrive at the best solution. Problems will occur as a nurse educator; our responsibility is to deal with them in a calm, professional, civil manner.

Be a duck.

PRINCIPLE

#4 Teamwork and collaboration is a QSEN competency that applies to nursing education at all levels.

Although it may not always be apparent, faculty and administrators are on the same team. Recently I was talking with the President of Academic Affairs at a college. The college is working on continuous quality improvement. My task was to review documents related to the nursing program faculty. Although most faculty are happy teaching in the nursing program, the administrator wants to discover what the administration can do to improve the nursing program. A task he especially wanted me to complete was a review of the nursing faculty handbook, college faculty contract, and any college level policies related to faculty to ensure they align with other nursing programs that I consider to be excellent. Then he shared that the driver of this project was student outcomes. The nursing program must improve student outcomes, especially the completion rate. His idea is, "happy faculty, successful students."

What the college does to support faculty has to be fair and reasonable to all parties. Faculty must give 100% to the nursing program and the college administration must be supportive of the nursing program while remaining fiscally responsible. Successful implementation of the roles of the members of these two professional classifications requires teamwork and collaboration.

There are times when it may seem faculty and administrators are working against one another. This is always a bothersome situation. Both faculty and administrators must have the same goals in mind, while respecting the vantage point and responsibilities of the other

> Teamwork and collaboration exist in nursing education as well as in nursing practice— or at least it should to achieve the best outcomes.

party. For satisfactory program outcomes to be achieved, all parties must work together knowing that each party must cooperate and collaborate. There is no place for hidden agenda with either faculty or administrators.

PRINCIPLE

#5 Orientation as a new faculty is important; know what you need to learn.

All faculty new to an academic setting need orientation and mentoring. Most state boards of nursing and nursing accreditation agencies require new faculty be oriented to their role within the nursing program. What that orientation entails varies depending on the needs of the faculty. If a new hire has experience in the faculty role, that person's needs are different than a new hire who has no experience in the academic setting.

Faculty need orientation to the institution as well as to the role of the academic nurse educator. It is helpful to have a checklist of topics covered during orientation. Obvious topics are those that explain the parent institution including college level policies, the organizational structure, and where nursing fits within the institution. Other obvious topics are those related to teaching in the various educational environments such as how to handle teaching in the classroom, clinical, skills laboratory, and simulation laboratory.

In my work as a nursing education consultant, there are some topics that often are not covered.

These topics include:

1. Regulatory approval. Most states have a Board of Nursing or other regulatory body such as a state education board that oversees most nursing programs. Some states require all types of nursing programs have regulatory approval and oversight. Other states only require regulatory oversight for pre-licensure programs and advanced practice (nurse practitioner) programs. Faculty should know which applies in the state in which they teach. Faculty should become very familiar with the rules and regulations of the regulatory body that oversees the nursing program.

2. Nursing accreditation. Which of the nursing accreditation agencies does the nursing program use? What is the faculty's role in the tasks required for accreditation? Does the program operate from an "accreditation ready" perspective? How does the program collect data, analyze data, trend data, and use data for ongoing program improvement as required for accreditation purposes?

3. The National Council of State Boards of Nursing (NCSBN). Faculty need to understand the function and purpose of the NCSBN. Faculty in all pre-licensure programs must have a good understanding of the research conducted by and documents published by the NCSBN and their importance to the programs in which they teach. All faculty should know what the detailed NCLEX Test Plans are and how they are used in their program. All faculty should know about the Practice Analysis and how to use it in their program. Finally, all pre-licensure programs should subscribe to their NCLEX Program Reports. These reports should be analyzed, discussed, and used for ongoing program improvement.

4. The program's systematic evaluation plan. Most state boards of nursing and all nursing accreditation bodies require the nursing program have a systematic evaluation plan. Faculty must learn about and participate in the tasks required to implement the systematic evaluation plan.

5. Faculty's job description. All faculty should be familiar with their job description. Each item on the job description has meaning. It is helpful to orient faculty about each item and what each item requires in terms of knowledge and job performance to complete all the tasks.

6. Faculty evaluation. It might seem obvious that faculty will be oriented to the evaluation process used, but I have worked with schools that do not have a specific process for evaluating faculty.

7. Faculty workload assignments. Workload assignments can be very confusing. Workload assignments should be fair and clearly explained. All faculty should understand how their workload is assigned including number of face-to-face teaching hours a week, office hours, preparation time, research requirements, time for committee work, and other workload factors.

8. Clinical agency contracts. If faculty teach in the clinical, it is critical they are familiar with what is in the contract signed by the college and the clinical agency. Typically, these contracts provide information about expectations of the school, the agency, the faculty, and the students while present in the clinical agency. Faculty are responsible for ensuring the terms of the contract are enforced and knowing the rights and responsibilities of all parties covered by the contract.

These are examples of topics that are often missing from new faculty orientation, but each is critical to a successful faculty experience. Review your school's orientation for new faculty to determine what might be missing.

The role of the academic nurse educator is multifaceted and so the orientation of new faculty should be multifaceted.

All faculty expectations— rights and responsibilities— should be clearly communicated.

PRINCIPLE
#6 Eat lunch with the new "kid."

Although this advice is widely applied to children, it also applies to faculty teaching in schools of nursing. It is important for new faculty to feel accepted and part of the group. So often we are distracted with so much to do—planning classes, engaging in research, grading papers, and on and on. We often forget there is a new faculty member until we have a faculty meeting. New faculty require mentoring—both formal and informal. Informal meetings over a quick cup of coffee are stimulating for both parties, not just from the caffeine but also from the collegiality and comradery developed during the meetings.

All faculty require mentoring—even if the newly hired faculty has experience teaching in other nursing programs. Newly hired faculty need to feel they fit in; they need to believe they are part of the group. They need to belong. Mentoring behaviors foster belongingness. The term belongingness refers to feeling essential, being an important part of something. Belongingness helps eliminate the perception of being on the fringe or marginalized resulting from feelings of not being accepted into the larger faculty group. All faculty are important.

> Newly hired faculty need to feel they fit in; they need to believe they are part of the group.
>
> Let's mentor new faculty—something that is good for both parties!

Be a mentor—even if informally over a cup of coffee.

Accepting Change

CHANGE IS INEVITABLE. The nursing profession and nursing practice change. Health care changes. Students change. The educational setting changes. Nursing education changes. However, the old saying, "The wheels of education turn slowly" often times applies to nursing education. Although much has changed in nursing education, such as online education and high-fidelity simulation, there is much that has not changed for decades.

Chapter 3 Principles

The Principles in this chapter demonstrate the importance of making changes when change is needed.

All chapters in this book, especially Chapter 4: Teaching and Learning Practices, discuss many areas of nursing education that need to change to improve the quality of nursing education. This chapter presents Principles specifically speaking to change itself.

As discussed in the introduction to Chapter 1: Who You Are as a Nurse Educator, consider change as it applies to your self-concept as a nurse educator. Do you accept change? Are you an early adopter of change; someone who waits to see if and how the change works, then adopts the change; or a never-changer. What messages does your self-concept give you about change? Does it say, "Let me consider this change and the data that support the change." Or, does your self-concept say, "This is the way I have always taught and see no reason to change now" or "This is the way I was taught in nursing school so I am going to teach the same as my teachers did."

The goal of the Principles in this chapter is to open minds to new ways of doing. Nursing educators cannot keep doing what has always been done when there is evidence that supports a need for change. One of faculty's overall responsibilities is to engage in ongoing program improvement. To meet that goal, change is often required. We cannot expect outcomes to improve if we do not change what we are doing.

PRINCIPLE

#1   Love what you do, but not how you do it.

In 1990, Alvin Toffler, the American writer and futurist, wrote:

> *The illiterate of the twenty-first century will not be*
> *those who cannot read and write,*
> *but those who cannot learn, unlearn, and relearn.*

This is so applicable to nursing education. Nursing education needs change, but when change is discussed, a major concern often comes in the form of the question: "How do you get faculty and others to accept a new way of doing? How can we get our faculty colleagues to understand that our decades old way of teaching needs to change?"

Unlearning is difficult. There is security in the known even if it isn't working. A very insightful book that talks about unlearning is *Higher Unlearning* (Uldrich, 2011). This book provides accounts about so many things that needed to be changed, but, even with solid evidence supporting the change, the changes took a very long time because people resisted the idea that the new was better. The book also makes the reader aware of the harm that can occur when change is not made regardless of the strong data to support the change.

The amount of work involved in learning a new way of doing, often with skepticism the new way will work, can solidify the resistance to change. This resistance to change is even present when there is evidence that current practices are not working.

Nursing education examples of areas that need change include:

1. The way we teach students to think.

2. The decades old approach to pre-licensure clinical education.

3. Expecting the completion of a 5-column care plan to demonstrate students can think using the nursing process.

4. Classroom approaches to teaching from heavy lecture to ways to apply thinking to the content.

The idea of unlearning a current way of doing, then learning a new way can be overwhelming, but is a necessary component to moving our nursing programs forward into the future rather than remaining stagnate by continuing to do what has been done in the past. We must always remember that we are teaching students for the future, not for the past.

Be willing to...
learn,
unlearn,
and relearn.

It is a good thing to love your work; it makes going to work a happy event. But we cannot be so entrenched in our current ways of doing that we are resistant to change. Love what you do, but not how you do it.

PRINCIPLE

#2 We cannot keep doing the same thing over and over and expect different results.

Why would we approach a teaching/learning problem in the same way, over and over, and expect different results? For over 40 years I have researched and studied how to teach students to think. For all those years and continuing today the major approach used in nursing education is this:

1. Give students patient situations in the form of case studies, simulation, or clinical patient assignments.

2. Ask questions.

3. Ask further probing questions.

4. Use Socratic questioning.

5. The more you do this, the better students will learn to "think like a nurse."

Consider the research about the abilities of newly licensed nurses to think based on this approach. The research reports that new graduates' ability to think is exceptionally poor even though all the participants in the study had passed the NCLEX and were licensed RNs (Kavanagh & Sharpnack, 2021). The NCSBN's research also demonstrated newly licensed nurses are not able to think at entry level expectations (Muntean, 2012). To address this flaw in measuring the newly graduated nurse's lack of thinking, the NCLEX underwent a major change to specifically measure clinical judgment.

Continuing to use this old approach to teaching thinking, but wrapping it in the new verbiage of the National Council's Clinical Judgment Measurement Model does not change the fact that the teaching (instructional strategies) is the same so the result will be no different. Students will think the way we teach them to think. If we do not like the way they are thinking, we need to teach them in a different way. To achieve better results with our efforts to teach thinking, the instructional strategies (teaching/learning strategies) must change. Again, we can't keep doing the same thing over and over and expect different results.

We must "drill down to the detail." We must **first** actually teach what clinical judgment is all about **THEN** we can require students to apply the detailed clinical judgment framework to guide their thinking to arrive at the answers to our probing questions (Caputi, 2022). Other Principles in this book provide specific information about how to better teach thinking (clinical judgment).

This example about not changing the way we teach students to think is just one example of resistance to change as mentioned in Principle #1.

Students will think the way
we teach them to think.

If we do not like the way
they are thinking,
we need to teach them
in a different way.

PRINCIPLE

#3   The most dangerous phrase in the nurse educator's language is, "We've always done it this way."

So many of the teaching/learning methodologies used in nursing education are based on "untested assumptions." Here are some examples:

1. Students must write care plans in the 5-column format to demonstrate they can use the nursing process to think like a nurse.

2. In clinical, students must provide total patient care for their assigned patients throughout most, if not all, of the nursing courses.

3. Most clinical "paperwork" should be done after clinical is over. Students should spend their time in clinical providing hands-on care, not completing homework assignments.

4. Faculty must grade clinical paperwork outside of clinical; there is no time in clinical to "grade papers."

5. We must cover a large amount of information in a course because students need all that information to pass the licensing exam.

6. Students cannot administer medications in the clinical if they do not score 100% on a dosage calculation test.

7. Unit exams should be 50 questions and final exams should be 75 questions.

These are some examples of doing what we have always done. We must think about, analyze, and study all that we do to determine if these practices are resulting in the best learning for students. We must look for new and better—more innovative— ways to teach nursing that result in better student learning outcomes. One way to do this is to read nursing education journals. There are excellent journals with

> Always be on the hunt for new, innovative, and better ways to teach.

columns that present nursing education research and innovative teaching strategies. Examples of these journals include *Nursing Education Perspectives, Nurse Educator, Journal of Nursing Education,* and *Teaching and Learning in Nursing* among others.

Always be on the hunt for new, innovative, and better ways to teach. Do not assume that the way we have always done something is the best, and only, way.

PRINCIPLE
#4   Consider new ways of doing.

In 2003, the National League for Nursing called on nurse educators to question the very nature of learning, teaching, and curriculum design in nursing education programs (NLN, 2003). Nurse educators were challenged to develop new ways of teaching in response to the rapidly changing healthcare environment.

Although this reference was published in 2003, innovation is needed more now than ever. Nurse educators are very innovative. Consider the very fast changes made during the Covid-19 pandemic. Nurse educators worked fast to create new ways to deliver the nursing curriculum. As the saying goes, necessity is the mother of invention, and Covid-19 forced nurse educators to invent. We must continue that spirit of innovation. The necessity to innovate is still there, although not as evident, or seemingly not as critical, as during the pandemic.

Once you innovate, share your innovation! Journals such as *Nurse Educator, Journal of Nursing Education,* and *Nursing Education Perspectives* have columns dedicated to publishing the innovative activities of nurse educators. Share what you innovate! Experiencing your manuscript published and your name in print is a great motivator to continue innovating!

As I wrote in the Introduction to this book, before an idea is considered a "brilliant idea," it often was considered a "crazy" idea. Be an innovator. I recall working with a school in 2007 to guide revision of their curriculum. At that time, I talked with them about writing end-of-program learning outcomes based on current nursing practice using research evidence and regulatory expectations for nurses. What the program teaches should be based on current practice.

This approach replaced the older approach of organizing the curriculum around a nursing theory. I also suggested writing more specific behavioral statements for learning outcomes—called competencies—so all faculty consistently measure student achievement of the learning outcomes. Some of the faculty at that time were resistant insisting they need to use a nurse theorist as their "conceptual framework."

Today, the accepted way to construct a nursing curriculum is to use learning outcomes and competencies based on what is needed for current practice (AACN, 2021). What appeared to be a crazy idea at THAT time is not only commonplace at this time, but an expectation.

Many brilliant ideas were once
considered crazy ideas.

PRINCIPLE

#5   How do you eat an elephant? One bite at a time!

During a recent discussion with a dean of a school of nursing, the dean shared their nursing program was in need of a curriculum revision. She stated their curriculum was over ten years old. She asked if I would be able to consult with her and the nursing program faculty to guide them through the curriculum revision process. She politely asked me NOT to use the term "curriculum revision." She stated that for faculty revising the curriculum was an overwhelming task and the term "curriculum revision" was a trigger for anxiety. It will be difficult for faculty to stick with the large task of curriculum revision and see it to completion.

To me, facing an overwhelming task reminds me of the saying:

How do you eat an elephant?

One bite at a time!

Start by dividing a large task into pieces; then break down each piece into smaller pieces and continue that process until the pieces are manageable. Once the pieces are of manageable size, plan when you will start and finish each task to ensure completion of the task based on your established timeline.

As you work through the large task of curriculum revision, identify ways each of those smaller "pieces" might be kept current on a continual basis so the curriculum is constantly updated in smaller pieces. This eliminates the need for a large curriculum revision in the future.

You can also apply this approach when tasked with academic work such as writing a dissertation. Many doctoral students finish all the course work for a doctoral degree, but never finish the dissertation. The dissertation is perceived to be such a huge, overwhelming task that many students just give up. Break down that dissertation into pieces. Focus on one piece at a time. Finish a piece then move on to the next piece. You may need to go back and revise earlier pieces, but accept that is part of the process. Keep it small; keep it bite-sized.

> A large overwhelming task
> is best handled in pieces.
>
> Completing smaller pieces
> provides a feeling of
> accomplishment and makes
> the larger task much
> more doable.

PRINCIPLE

#6

The status quo should never be good enough—always seek to improve your own performance and the performance of your students.

Quality improvement matters. Think "upstream" to continuously improve before the need to improve becomes a necessity. For example, pre-licensure nursing programs prepare students to take the NCLEX. The NCLEX measures the candidates' knowledge of content and how to use that content in a nursing situation by applying clinical judgment. The NCSBN conducts research every three years to determine what changes might be made on the NCLEX based on current practice. Revisions that are made include changes to the detailed objectives and the percent of questions from each major area on the NCLEX test plan. The NCSBN also makes a decision about the passing standard which reflects the difficulty of the test items. They determine if the passing standard should remain at the current level or if it should be raised because new graduates are required to think at higher levels. The higher the level of thinking as revealed by their research, the more difficult the test items become.

When the passing standard is raised, schools work to determine how they can help improve their students' level of thinking to meet the increased expectations of NCLEX. Thinking upstream in this situation means always teaching students how to think at a higher-level of thinking **before** the passing standard is raised. Faculty should always teach students to think at the highest possible level regardless of the passing standard set by the NCSBN. For that reason,

> The status quo should never be good enough—no matter how good the status quo is.

my mantra has always been, "Teach students to think at such a high level, NCLEX will have to catch up with you!" This is one way to think upstream to continuously improve the quality of your nursing program.

Teaching and Learning Practices

THE CORE OF THE NURSE EDUCATOR'S roles and responsibilities is to teach so students will learn. What that means varies greatly among faculty because the teaching/learning process is multifaceted. Some factors that affect the teaching/learning process include student characteristics, the curriculum, the level of nurse being educated, prior teaching experience, institutional support for faculty, institutional support for students, the nursing program budget, and the facilities in which students learn. Considering this list is not all-inclusive, it is apparent the educator's teaching involves a high level of skill, knowledge, and confidence.

The 40 principles in this chapter only touch on some of these factors. The goal of this chapter is to stimulate thinking and conversations among faculty. Some of the content may be familiar to faculty, but some of the content may be somewhat foreign and even difficult for some faculty to accept.

Hopefully, faculty read these Principles together then engage in thoughtful conversation about how they might be used in the nursing program.

Chapter 4 Principles

The Principles in this chapter provide best practices in teaching/learning in nursing education.

Many current practices are built on false assumptions; that is, we assume this is what we need to do because this is what we have always done.

These Principles look at some of those old practices and provide new practices to replace them.

PRINCIPLE

#1 Develop an evidence-based, competency-based nursing curriculum.

Competency-based nursing education has been used for decades. Many nursing education programs have developed competency-based curricula. A competency-based curriculum is one that develops general learning outcomes, then for each learning outcome, develops specific, measurable competencies (behaviors incorporating knowledge, skills, values, and attitudes) that are used to assess student achievement of each learning outcome. AACN (2021) defines competencies as:

> "An observable ability of a health professional, integrating multiple components such as knowledge, skills, values, and attitudes. Since competencies are observable, they can be measured and assessed to ensure their acquisition" (p. 56).

A set of competencies for each learning outcome makes clear what is expected of the student to achieve the learning outcome. AACN suggests using competencies to delineate student behaviors that are expected and measurable to achieve each of the learning outcomes. This provides consistency among faculty about student expectations.

The following provides additional information about competencies:

- Learning outcomes are broad statements and the competencies for each learning outcome delineate the specific behaviors the student must achieve to demonstrate achievement of the learning outcome. Successfully performing each of the competencies (expectations) demonstrates the student has attained the learning outcome.

- Competency statements are used to assess and evaluate each student's achievement of the learning outcomes.

- Faculty identify at what level and in what manner students will achieve the competencies in each course.

- Bloom's taxonomy is used to level both the learning outcomes and the competencies from course to course as they build across the program to culminate in the program learning outcomes and competencies.

To write competencies for each learning outcome, faculty engage in the following curriculum activities.

1. Start with writing program learning outcomes based on evidence from the nursing education and nursing practice literature about expectations of the newly graduated nurse. Consider national guidelines to use to develop the program learning outcomes, then determine what competencies demonstrate achievement of each learning outcome.

2. Develop course learning outcomes and competencies based on the program learning outcomes and competencies.

3. Not all program **learning outcomes** need to be reflected in every course. The **learning outcomes** for a specific course depend on the focus of the course.

4. Not all the **competencies** for each learning outcome need to be included in every course. The **competencies** for each learning outcome for a specific course depend on the focus of the course.

5. The competencies (like the learning outcomes) stay consistent across the program courses, but are leveled from course to course and address the major focus of the course (pediatric, adult health, public health, etc.). Eventual achievement of the **program** learning outcomes and competencies depends on student achievement of the learning outcomes and competencies of **each course** as they build across the program.

So where do faculty locate evidence-based competencies? It is important to note that if faculty are creating an evidence-based curriculum, more than one source of competencies is used. The American Association of Colleges of Nursing has published many competencies in their *Essentials* document. I caution faculty from using just this one document as the sole source of competencies. Faculty should reference other evidence-based documents as they develop the program learning outcomes and competencies.

Some of these sources include:

- *The Essentials: Core Competencies for Professional Nursing Education* (American Association of Colleges of Nursing, 2021).

- *Outcomes and Competencies for Graduates of Practical/Vocational, Diploma, Associate Degree, Baccalaureate, Master's, Practice Doctorate, and Research Doctorate Programs in Nursing* (National League for Nursing, 2012).

- Quality and Safety Education for Nurses (QSEN.org).

- The Detailed NCLEX Test Plans (NCSBN, 2023).

- *Nursing Scope and Standards of Practice*, (ANA, 2021).

- *NLN Core Competencies for Nurse Educators* (Halstead, 2019) for developing a curriculum for a graduate level nurse educator program.

- Your state nurse practice act for scope of practice of the level of nurse the program is educating.

- Discussions with your local healthcare agencies. These discussions are critical to determine what is occurring in local practice.

Many of these sources become dated and may not totally represent current practice when you are ready to revise your curriculum. For example, the *Essentials* document was revised in 2021, but the previous version was dated 2008. The NLN's *Outcomes and Competencies* document is dated 2012.

All the above documents are used as well as others such as documents with competencies for specific practice areas for nurse practitioners to develop those graduate curricula. Evidence-based nursing education requires using evidence-based practice documents to develop nursing curricula at all levels.

Competency-based education is touted as academia's solution to decrease the ever-growing education-to-practice gap (Wittmann-Price & Gittings, 2021). It is important for faculty to contemplate just what that means.

Here are other factors that need to be considered when developing a competency-based curriculum.

- What exactly are the gaps between academia and practice? These are not clearly defined. If they are defined, they may be from a regional or national perspective and not include local considerations important for your graduates.

- Does the total responsibility to close those gaps lie solely with academia or should practice also be involved?

- Just writing a competency-based curriculum does not address the education-to-practice gap without practice and academia working together. Practice must identify expectations of new graduates and academia must discuss what is actually possible. What academia can achieve in the education of nurses is limited by several factors. These include the limitation of credit hours and length of time in the program. Some nursing programs may also be limited by the type of student experiences available in the clinical setting. For example, some clinical agencies do not allow students access to the electronic medical record. If lack of technology skills is part of the education-to-practice gap, this clinical limitation needs to be addressed.

Once the details of the perceived education-to-practice gap are identified, some of the gaps may be achieved while students are enrolled in a nursing program, but some may need to be included as part of the orientation program provided by the healthcare agency. Practice and academic should work together to determine which partner does what.

Competency-based curricula have been used for many years, but issues still persist such as the widening education-to-practice gap. The answer is to build an evidence-based, competency-based nursing curriculum taking into consideration the factors listed above.

Faculty must also determine how the competency-based curriculum will be implemented. Prior to developing an evidence-based, competency-based nursing program curriculum, faculty should discuss how to implement such a curriculum then, once in place, ensure the curriculum is consistently implemented as intended for the best results from the competency-based curriculum.

> Competency-based education
> is not new, but has become
> the preferred method for
> developing nursing curricula
> by using program and course
> outcomes and competencies.

PRINCIPLE

#2   It's all about consistency.

All faculty should implement the curriculum and all its components—including teaching/learning strategies and test item writing—in a consistent manner across the nursing program.

A very big weakness that I see across all levels of nursing education and across the country is lack of a consistent approach for delivering the curriculum and all its components. A perfect example of this is how we teach students to think like a nurse. Nursing education has always struggled with teaching students to think, and I believe one of the major issues is a lack of consistency in teaching what thinking is then applying a specific thinking process to nursing content across the curriculum.

I was once hired by a Vice President of Academic Affairs. He explained the nursing program is in need of help because of low completion rates and low NCLEX pass rates. I reviewed a lot of the documents of the nursing program then visited the campus. When it was time for me to meet with the nursing faculty, I realized all my interaction to date were with upper-level administration and very little with those in the nursing program. When I met with faculty, I asked them why they thought I was there and what I could do for them.

The nursing program plan of study included two years of nursing courses. A group of faculty taught the first year of nursing courses and another group taught the second year of nursing courses. A faculty member who taught in the second year of the nursing courses spoke up immediately. She shared with me and the group that the problem is that students enter the second year of nursing courses not knowing how to think because they were not taught to think in the first year. Therefore, the students struggle with the higher-cognitive level test items in the second year and have difficulty applying thinking to patient care.

After she spoke, there was a short pause. Then a faculty member for the first-year nursing courses responded. She said, "If you think students don't know how to think when they get to the second year of nursing courses, you should have seen them when they came in! You're lucky we got them that far!"

It was immediately clear this was not a student issue or a faculty issue—it was a curriculum issue! I had reviewed the curriculum prior to my campus visit. There was very little indication that students were actually taught a process for thinking. There was nothing that explained at what level of thinking the students should be at the end of each semester, how they got to that level, and the assessment measures to determine student achievement. Every faculty determined on their own how they would teach and evaluate thinking. There was no consistency among faculty.

This is what happens when there is not a consistent approach to delivering the curriculum. All faculty do the best they can to teach what they think they should be teaching, but their approaches all differ. Faculty often are inconsistent in the way content is taught and applied. Without program policies on how to deliver the curriculum, every faculty is determining for themselves what to do and how to do it. Students then spend their time determining how each faculty teaches and tests rather than building on what they previously learned and how they learned to think.

I strongly suggest adopting a program-wide approach about how to deliver the curriculum in the nursing classroom and clinical setting. A consistent approach provides students reassurance that they do not have to adjust to a different way of teaching with each new nursing course. This also provides faculty with critical information about how students learned in previous nursing courses which strengthens the current faculty's effectiveness. Inconsistencies in teaching leave faculty unsure how students have engaged with content in previous nursing courses. It's all about consistency.

> A consistent approach to
> delivering a curriculum has the
> best chances for success.

PRINCIPLE

#3 Know where what you are teaching fits into the overall curriculum.

It's all about the program learning outcomes! Academic accreditation agencies and regulatory bodies such as the state boards of nursing require educational programs to measure their students' achievement of program learning outcomes. All nursing courses in the program plan of study contribute to the end-of-program learning outcomes.

In my role as a nursing education consultant and as an accreditation site visitor, I would ask faculty: "Tell me how what you teach in your assigned nursing courses expands on the nursing courses students completed prior to this term and prepares them for the courses in subsequent terms." Many times, the answer was, "I do not know. I have never taught those courses."

This is an outdated way of doing. We no longer teach just a certain content area without any connection to the prerequisite courses or with no knowledge about the courses in subsequent terms. This may be why students have difficulty recalling what they previously learned. The courses we teach and how we teach them are all part of the bigger picture. We must support previous learning by requiring students to actively recall and apply that learning to what they are learning in the current course.

All the general concepts of a nursing program connect. For example, if students learn about the concept of pain in fundamentals, they apply that concept to the care of all patients. When caring for a patient who just delivered a baby, the nurse addresses the concept of pain in the care of that patient. Students can compare and contrast the assessment data and treatment of pain for the postpartum patient with patients they cared for in a previous course such as an elderly patient in pain or a postoperative patient in pain. Comparing and contrasting nursing care of various types of patients expands the student's understanding of the concept of pain and how interventions to treat pain are the same and how they are different depending on the individual patient situation. Students learn to use situation-based thinking (advanced beginner thinking) rather than rule-based thinking (novice level thinking). This type of learning activity is critical as the student learns clinical judgment.

This overall Principle of "Know where what you are teaching fits into the overall curriculum" translates to: No more teaching in silos. We all contribute to the developing nurse our curriculum is preparing. Success as a faculty is measured by evaluating not just students' achievement of the course learning outcomes, but also their achievement of the end-of-program learning outcomes. For that reason, we must know where what we are teaching fits into the overall curriculum.

No more teaching in silos.

PRINCIPLE

#4 Teaching too much content can interfere with student success.

For decades we have heard about the bloated curriculum. Faculty often fear not teaching students everything faculty believe the students should know. However, most nursing programs do not have a program-wide policy faculty use to determine what content to teach and what content not to teach.

Expecting students to learn too much content by assigning hundreds of pages of textbook readings and completing assignments from numerous other resources does not contribute to student success. Students may have these types of heavy assignments in every nursing course they are taking in a term. Students are not able to complete all these assignments even if they devoted all their outside-of-class time in an attempt to complete all that is assigned. Nursing curricula are bloated and require students to learn too much. The end result is students try to prioritize the homework assignments without any basis for how to do so. Students typically are on their own with this prioritization exercise. Both students and faculty become frustrated—students because they cannot complete all the assigned work and faculty because students do not complete all the assigned work. The bottom line is faculty must cut content.

I believe most faculty would love to cut content but they just do not have the confidence for doing so. They may worry that faculty in subsequent courses will complain students do not know something those faculty believe the students should have learned in prior terms. Another issue is faculty do not have a process to guide them on content selection and deletion. So, what might you do?

To start the process of cutting content, make sure you teach the "need to know" and cut down on the extra material that is the "nice to know." To make that differentiation consider the following:

1. Teach what is actually happening in practice. Compare what is in the curriculum and student assignments to what nurses do in practice. For example, do nurses complete 5-column care plans in practice? How do they use the nursing process throughout the day?

Can faculty replace the care plans with the way nurses actually use the nursing process? This is one example, look for others in your curriculum.

2. Delete content that is not in the "commonly occurring" category; only focus on common disorders and diseases. For example, for renal cover topics such as renal failure, calculi, and other common conditions. Do not teach conditions such as pheochromocytoma. Look to reliable resources for incidence of diseases. If it is a rare disease, do not teach it even if it is in the textbook. For example, the National Institute of Diabetes and Digestive and Kidney Disease reports that diabetes insipidus is a rare disorder so might be one you do not cover in your curriculum. Addison's disease is considered uncommon according to Mayoclinic.org so you may choose not to teach Addison's disease.

3. Teach only the **most commonly prescribed** medications. Faculty may want to access the 200 most commonly prescribed medications published by the National Library of Medicine at: https://www.ncbi.nlm.nih.gov/pmc/articles/PMC6025009/. Depending on the level of nurse the program is preparing, it may not be necessary to teach all 200. When teaching students drug classifications, it would be prudent to use this list to select associated medications. This list is subject to change as the drug market changes and new research is published, so faculty will want to access it frequently for any updates.

4. Use other credible websites to determine what is most important to teach. Consult the Centers for Disease Control's "Number of deaths for leading causes of death" report. In December, 2022, the list of leading causes of death in order of highest to lowest included:

    i.   Heart disease
    ii. Cancer
    iii. COVID-19
    iv. Accidents (unintentional injuries)
    v.   Stroke (cerebrovascular diseases)

   vi.   Chronic lower respiratory diseases

   vii.   Alzheimer's disease

   viii.   Diabetes

   ix.   Influenza and pneumonia

   x.   Nephritis, nephrotic syndrome, and nephrosis

This list of common causes of death is updated yearly so faculty will want to review the site often. Suicide has always been included in the 10 leading causes of death. However, recently suicide is not on the top ten list likely because of the addition of Covid-19. As death rates drop from Covid-19, the list will change.

The CDC also tracks causes of death for specific groups. Faculty should monitor other areas of the CDC website which report causes of death by sex, race, and minority groups. The causes of death for those groups of people may be somewhat different than leading causes of death for the general population.

5. For pre-licensure nursing programs review the latest practice analysis from the National Council of State Boards of Nursing. These reports provide direction on how much content in various areas of practice should be included in the nursing curriculum. These reports provide valuable information to direct nursing curricula.

6. Consult other credible websites dedicated to specific populations of patients. For example, look to the National Alliance for Mental Illness (NAMI) for common mental health illnesses. Faculty may also refer to the Association of Women's Health, Obstetric, and Neonatal Nurses (AWHONN) website for priority issues for this population to include in the curriculum. The Institute of Pediatric Nursing provides child health statistics that can be used to determine priority pediatric issues. There are a number of reliable resources that provide information for the aging population. One such resource is the NIH's National Institute on Aging. A focus on patients 65 years and older should be a priority in both Registered Nursing and Practical/Vocational Nursing programs. The NCSBN Practice Analysis for both RNs and LPN/VNs confirms the majority group of patients for whom new graduates provide care is 65 years and older.

7. The above resources provide national data about important topics to teach. You must also consider local topics. For this information, check with your local healthcare agencies where students enjoy clinical experiences. Survey the unit managers in the emergency department and the obstetric, pediatric, medical, surgical, mental health, and other units about the most common illnesses and healthcare problems cared for in their agencies. Common conditions and diseases may emerge that are not on the national lists. It would be important to include any of these commonly seen healthcare concerns in those agencies because students will care for these patients.

8. Finally, do not teach two curricula by teaching: (i) your program curriculum as approved by your regulatory agency and your accreditation body, and (ii) the curriculum of a standardized testing company. The curriculum nursing faculty assemble should be what is needed for your graduates to be successful on a licensing exam, on a certification exam, and in practice. Requiring students to learn two curricula overwhelms and frustrates students. In my discussions with students, they report they do not know what to do first. Some students question why they need a second curriculum. Requiring students to learn what is necessary for the program's curriculum and for a second curriculum developed by a standardized testing company has further bloated the curriculum at a time when the call—which has been out for decades—is to decrease content in the nursing curriculum and make room for active application of clinical judgment to content taught in each course.

Teaching too much content can interfere with student success. This Principle calls upon faculty to provide as much evidence as possible when selecting the "most important" content to teach. As faculty, we often get caught up in the topics we love to teach (I know I did!) and end up teaching too much content. Help your students succeed by cutting content. For the nursing curriculum, more is not necessarily better.

> Decrease the amount of content taught to achieve desirable NCLEX pass rates and completion rates.

PRINCIPLE

#5 Teach resilience—a term fairly new to nursing education.

Nursing has always been very demanding, exhausting work. Nurses rarely experience "an easy day at work." There is always so much going on, so many things to think about, so many patients depending on the nurse for their very safety. And that's the normal course of events. When an unexpected event occurs, the nurse must remain calm, remain in charge, and make clear, accurate decisions. This describes resiliency.

Sieg (2020) defines resilience as "the capacity to accurately perceive and respond well to stressful situations" (para. 2). Our students must learn to be resilient. We must include the study of resilience and mindfulness in our curriculum. We must provide students instruction on how to stay calm and focus their thinking to make the best decisions possible in a stressful situation.

There is a connection between learning clinical judgment and becoming resilient (Caputi, 2022). You can learn more about this connection at https://lindacaputi.com/blog/ and read my blog titled "Resiliency and Clinical Judgment—What's the connection?" Using a clinical judgment framework to guide their thinking helps students and new graduates to stay mindful, resilient, and in control of the situation. Nurses need this training for the safety of their patients, but also for their own mental health. We must incorporate resiliency training into our programs.

> There is a connection between learning clinical judgment and becoming resilient.

PRINCIPLE

#6 The iGen students are not the first generation of students who do not read.

In my consulting work, I often hear: "This generation of students does not read." To some extent, this is true. Because of those little electronic devices, information is readily available, albeit in brief format. The information is even available without reading. Using our voice to ask one of the electronic intelligence assistants (such as Siri) a question, we get a verbal answer— like magic!

However, because the current generation of students (also known as the iGen generation) was raised with easy access to information does not make them unique as the first generation of students who "do not read before coming to class." Students not reading has always been a major complaint from faculty. I recall listening to Dr. Nancy Diekelmann (Professor Emerita at the University of Wisconsin-Madison School of Nursing) at a conference in the early 2000s. She shared with the audience that research at that time showed that even the A students do not read before attending class. The conclusion was that faculty required very heavy reading assignments that often were not realistic or ever referenced in class or tested on exams. Students reported they would attend class, take notes about what the faculty discussed, then read those sections of the text that related to what was discussed in class.

Perhaps the issue is not that students do not read, but that reading assignments are too broad, too general, and too much. We must make reading assignments purposeful. All homework must be purposeful!

Bernard, Rosales, and Zurcher (2022) conducted research to explore students' motivation to prepare for class. Their research revealed that when students have worksheets to complete prior to class and are called upon in class to use information from those worksheets, students are motivated to complete the homework. As one student noted, the worksheets provided direction about what was important to study.

Students want direction for what to study and to know their study time is purposeful. Learning is deeper and more lasting when it is effortful (Brown, Roediger, & McDaniel, 2014). The worksheets take effort to complete and require effort when students are asked to connect what is on the worksheets to classroom learning. Learning is deeper and more lasting when it is both meaningful and effortful.

Perhaps the issue is not that
students do not read,
but that reading assignments
are too broad, too general,
and too much.

We must make reading
assignments purposeful.

PRINCIPLE

#7 Ensure the reading level of the required textbooks is at or below the reading ability of your students.

In my consulting work with schools, I often ask students about their textbooks. It is common for students to share they do not read their textbooks because they have difficulty understanding what the book is saying. Students have shared their experiences, such as: "I read the fundamentals book because I can understand it. I don't read the med/surg book because it is too difficult to understand."

Students are sometimes required to read assignments from nursing textbooks they are not able to understand. The text may use high-level English language which students are not able to process. Or, many students who are English Language Learners may find the level of English in the textbooks a challenge. This lack of ability to process some textbooks is not a reflection of the students' ability to learn. Rather, it reflects a challenge for faculty to select textbooks that best meet the needs of the students.

Nursing language and medical terminology are foreign to students, so they are reading textbooks that are challenging to process as well as learning a new language. This is especially problematic for students in nursing programs where nursing courses start in the first or second term of the entire program plan of study. For these programs, students have little experience reading college level textbooks even though they may be required to take some prerequisite courses prior to enrolling in nursing courses.

It is always best to determine the reading level of textbooks through your own means. You can cut and paste a passage from the book into an application such as Word* to obtain a reading level of that passage. You might also ask one of your English faculty to determine the reading level.

It is also important to seek **student** input prior to selecting textbooks. Students are the end users of the texts. If they find a textbook difficult to process, there is no reason to require that text regardless of how much the faculty believe the text is useful. In the Appendices of this book, I provide the *Textbook Evaluation Tool* which I developed and have used many times. You might consider using that tool to guide your selection of textbooks. Note there is a section at the end of the tool that seeks student input.

> It is important to seek **student** input prior to selecting textbooks.

PRINCIPLE

#8 Always make homework assignments doable and meaningful.

The "Old Days" of Homework in Nursing Education

The "old days" refers to the traditional way of assigning homework. The process for assigning homework was something like this:

- Consider the topics students are to learn each week.

- Assign chapters from the textbook on those topics.

- Assign other homework based on the electronic resources from the textbook, online videos, podcasts, or materials from a standardized testing company.

- Ask students to complete all the assignments then be prepared for class discussion.

That was pretty much it! But what does "be prepared" mean? How will students know they are prepared for class? How will faculty assess students' readiness for class?

The "New Days" of Homework in Nursing Education

As previously mentioned in another Principle, faculty have shared that "students do not read before they come to class." This applies to all "generations" of learners, not just the iGen students now entering college who are accustomed to reading short texts, messages from their friends in group chats, or watching short online videos.

The movement to the "flipped classroom" that started about 15 years ago encouraged students to work through content in some meaningful way prior to arriving at class. Classroom time was focused on application of the material to various contexts. No "lecture"—totally application in the classroom. For some this "no lecture" approach was too extreme for both students and faculty.

A newer trend is the "scrambled classroom." In the scrambled classroom, throughout the class session faculty deliver short bursts of lecture to discuss harder to understand material or material students typically struggle with, or to clarify student questions. Active learning is also used intermittently during the class time. Faculty presentation and active learning are intermixed throughout the class time.

Regardless of which approach is used for classroom learning, homework assignments must change. The most difficult aspect of changing an approach to assigning homework is the idea of change itself. It may be difficult for nursing faculty to change. Both seasoned (experienced) and new nursing faculty struggle with change. Experienced faculty may say, "But this is the way I do it and it works." Faculty new to education may say, "But this is the way I learned in nursing school." These are not reasons to continue using the old way of assigning homework. It is clear that homework assignments in pre-licensure nursing programs are out of control and typically not very meaningful or helpful.

Some Guidelines for Planning Homework

No one likes homework—neither students nor faculty. Faculty do not like assigning homework because there is always the fear students will not complete the homework. Students do not like homework for a number of reasons, but one reason is there is too much! Students often ask themselves a number of questions such as:

1. How will I ever finish all the homework?

2. What homework assignments are most important?

3. What if I do all the homework and it is never mentioned in class? Will that be a waste of my time?

4. Should I do the homework from the course textbook for the class or the homework to prepare for the standardized test I will take next week?

Students should not have these or other questions when deciding what homework assignments to complete. All homework assignments should be doable and meaningful. All homework should be purposeful. Students should know the homework will be used in class, and students should know the homework will be needed when taking the course exams.

Faculty should review the homework assigned to determine if:

1. Student time is well spent on the homework assignments.

2. The time required to complete all the homework assignments is fair and reasonable.

3. The time students are spending has a return on their investment in terms of learning—and, yes, in terms of preparing for the class exam.

Students often have a limited amount of time to engage in homework assignments. It is important faculty only assign homework that is **purposeful**. Students are responsible for doing the homework, but **faculty are responsible for realistic homework expectations and assigning homework that is doable and meaningful**.

Students must be held accountable for completing homework assignments. Faculty can assess if homework is completed by requiring students to use the materials during class time. This gives the student a reason to do the homework. When calling on students to use the homework in class, faculty can determine which students are completing the homework and which students are not. Faculty can then consult with those who are not. However, assign too much homework and there is a high probability students will not complete the homework.

Additionally, students should see a direct and clear connection between the homework activities and questions on the classroom exam. That is the students' ultimate payoff for completing the homework—a direct connection to what they will need to know when taking the exam.

Summary

- Plan homework with a **purpose**. The homework should involve preparation of materials needed to engage students in active learning activities in the classroom, apply content to nursing practice, and engage in higher level thinking.

- Simplify homework assignments. Develop and assign homework sheets with fill-in-the blank information students will reference in the classroom for application of the reading material to classroom activities.

- Homework focuses on content; in-class activities focus on using clinical judgment to connect homework content to specific patient scenarios. In class application of clinical judgment role models clinical judgment as the bridge between content and application to individual patient situations.

- Link the homework to activities in class and to what will be on the exam including the type of test items students will answer. This applies to both content and thinking. Here is the flow:

  > Complete and bring homework sheets to class → Students actively relate the content in homework assignments to what is discussed in class and apply clinical judgment to case studies → Students work through in-class practice test questions based on homework assignments while applying clinical judgment using NCLEX-style testing → Actual exam items structured the same as the in-class practice questions but using different content than what was used in the classroom.

- Students should experience the faculty role modeling the detailed clinical judgment framework they are learning in the first term applied to content, then used to answer test items. See the various Principles in this section on teaching clinical judgment.

- All faculty must use the language of a detailed clinical judgment framework to role model how clinical judgment is the bridge— the bridge that connects classroom content to individual patient situations.

Homework focuses on content;
in-class activities focus on
using clinical judgment to
connect homework content to
specific patient scenarios.

PRINCIPLE
#9   Guide students through their homework.

Faculty often assign students to watch pre-recorded lectures as their homework. Students should be actively involved with these pre-recorded lectures and not passively watch and listen to the speaker. In the recording faculty connect what they are discussing to the reading assignments. Students are instructed to pause, read some material in the book, restart the recording to listen to faculty expanding on the content, then again pause the recording to complete the homework sheets that will be used in class.

During the recording faculty can explain what parts of the reading assignment are important and what pages of the chapters do not need to be read. The recording should help students sort through all the information in the text and focus on what is important to learn at that point in the curriculum. There is much information in textbooks students do not need to read. Pointing out what to read and what not to read is very helpful in these homework recordings.

It is very beneficial to guide students as they work through their homework. Pre-recordings are a great way to provide that benefit.

There is much information in
textbooks students do
not need to read.

Guide students through
their homework readings.

PRINCIPLE

#10 Students should fail themselves; they should get no help from faculty.

Faculty often fear it may be their fault if a student fails. I understand that fear and experienced it myself. An important principle in education is that if students fail, they should do so on their own with no help from faculty. But how can you ensure this will always be the case?

The best way to prevent contributing to a student's failure is to ensure quality education. Here are some suggestions:

1. Only teach content that is necessary.

2. Determine a reasonable amount of content for students to learn based on the credit hours assigned to your course.

3. Provide quality, active, engaged teaching/learning in the classroom.

4. Be available to answer questions and help students process content. Students should not be told faculty are too busy to work with them.

5. Ensure all assessment tools, including exams and clinical evaluation tools, are valid and reliable.

6. Provide individualized, teacher-guided remediation to help students who perform poorly on an exam or other assessment tool. Students need help filling in the gaps of the content they did not learn. They need help learning to think at the cognitive level required of the course. That remediation should be provided close to the assessment event and be directed by the faculty.

7. For each student who does not score 80% or higher on an exam, meet one-on-one with the student to review the exam and provide guidance. The guidance should fill in knowledge gaps, gaps in thinking ability, and test-taking strategies. Consider using the Exam Analysis Tool developed by faculty at Loma Linda University. Refer to the Appendices for a copy of this tool or access the tool at: https://lindacaputi.com/teaching-tools/.

Continue to add to this list with your own course-specific interventions for helping students succeed.

> The best way to prevent
> contributing to a student's
> failure is to ensure
> quality education.

PRINCIPLE

#11 Know your audience.

Know your audience is a basic principle of public speaking. You must speak to the needs and wants of your audience. This speaking principle is easily revised to apply to teaching—know your students.

As I work with schools across the country, I continue to learn that all nursing students are not the same and that students change over time. Student characteristics vary across program types and across the many different areas of this vast country. It is important to know your student characteristics and plan learning activities accordingly. Generational characteristics, grade point average, prior experience with college level courses, status as a first-generation college student, abilities in reading and math, grasp of the English language, and family/work responsibilities are some of the various characteristics to consider.

Consider two groups of students:

1. Group 1: The average GPA of this group is 3.8. Characteristics of these students include: full-time student status; not married; live on campus; parents are alumni of the college; average age is 21; not employed in a job; completed all non-nursing courses prior to entering the nursing sequence of courses.

2. Group 2: The average GPA of this group is 2.9. Characteristics of these students include: part-time student status; single parent or married with children; employed 20 to 30 hours a week; first generation college student; average age is 29; English is not their primary language; taking non-nursing courses while enrolled in nursing courses.

Faculty's approach teaching these two groups of students would be—and should be—very different. It is critical that faculty consider both academic and non-academic factors about their students when developing an approach to teaching and learning activities. Both groups of students can be successful, but their success is directly related to how faculty use these student characteristics to plan teaching/learning activities.

The literature is full of information about "traditional" and "non-traditional" nursing students. I suggest not using these labels. Non-traditional students may represent a collective majority in many nursing programs. Using the labels leads to assumptions that may or may not apply to your particular group of students. Additionally, these labels and their presumed definitions have been used for decades. Student characteristics are fluid and change over time. Student characteristics change about every 10 years with many changes related to societal issues. The teaching/learning processes used by faculty 10 years ago may no longer work with the current population of students.

It is best for faculty to describe their students' characteristics and address what can be done to meet their specific needs rather than assign a label and work from the label. Know your students and their characteristics. Teaching/learning practices must be designed to meet the students' specific needs. Just as nurses provide individualized, patient-centered care, faculty should provide individualized, student-centered education.

Plan teaching practices
based on the characteristics
of **your** students.

PRINCIPLE

#12   Identify pain points in your nursing program.

The term "pain point" first appeared in 1986. This business term is used to identify problems that result in frequent inconveniences or annoyances for customers. Businesses with an established market can identify pain points of that market and work to correct issues causing them.

Pain points are now being identified in health care. For example, in December, 2021, the New Jersey State Nurses Association conducted a survey to determine pain points for staff nurses (https://njsna.org/nurses-share-pain-points/). That survey reports that:

- Nearly 37% of nurses identify as being burned out, stressed, and/or overworked.

- 32% of nurses are very/completely satisfied with their occupation, compared to 52% prior to the Covid-19 pandemic.

- 29% of nurses say their desire to leave the profession is dramatically higher now versus pre-pandemic, noting the nursing shortage and inadequate staffing levels as top contributors to the low satisfaction.

- 66% of nurses expressed some level of consideration to leave the profession, signaling long-term impacts on the health system post-pandemic.

Healthcare organizations can use this information to determine if these are pain points in their individual institutions and, if so, identify and correct the causes.

Nursing education might also use this process. What are pain points for your nursing students? Here are some possible pain points:

- Faculty not available to answer student questions.

- Not enough parking. Seems petty, but if the students can't find a place to park, they often arrive late to class and that creates an additional pain point.

- Paying for required materials that are not used in the nursing program.

- Exams that somehow just don't make sense to them.

- Faculty who give the impression they do not care about the students' well-being.

- Unclear policies or policies inconsistently applied to students.

Nursing faculty and nursing program administrators have created many ways to identify pain points their students may be experiencing. They use informal meetings such as "Coffee with the Dean" hour, faculty office hours designated for discussions with students as a group or individually, and end-of-course evaluations.

Although these data collection activities have been in place for some time, the data may not have been aggregated, trended, and used to make changes to eliminate the pain points for future students. It is always better to prevent issues that cause annoyances than to deal with them in real time. Keeping issues to a minimum is helpful for the best use of student and faculty time and to establish an environment for success.

> It is always better to prevent issues that cause annoyances than to deal with them in real time.

Use the data to identify your pain points and proactively make changes.

PRINCIPLE

#13 Nursing program admission criteria need to be fair and reliable.

The purpose of admission criteria is to determine if the applicant is prepared to do well in nursing courses. Admission criteria are used to determine the student's readiness for successful completion of nursing courses in the first term. Admission criteria should be data driven based on evidence the criteria are reliable indicators of the student's ability to be successful in the nursing program.

There are two important aspects to consider related to admission criteria. The first is that admission criteria must be fair. I have worked with some schools that require students to take a standardized test that covers a number of content areas that are not required as pre-requisites to entering the program or may not be required as part of the nursing program plan of study. Yet, the students' composite scores are ranked and students are awarded points for the score they earned.

For example, the nursing program does not require a chemistry course. However, the composite score on the standardized exam includes a score on a chemistry portion of the exam. Although not required, some students may have taken chemistry and therefore score higher and have a better chance of being selected for acceptance into the program. This represents an unfair advantage for the student who has taken a chemistry course over a student who has not taken a chemistry course, although a chemistry course is not required for the nursing program.

All evaluation methods used before and during a nursing program should be fair, including evaluating methods used to determine admission into a nursing program.

The second important aspect of admission criteria is reliability. Any admission criteria used should be vetted as reliable indicators the student is academically prepared to do well in the first term of nursing courses. For each student, the level of achievement on each criterion should be recorded. Grades earned in all the first term nursing courses should then be recorded. Faculty can compare and contrast the admission criteria data with the grades in the nursing courses to determine if the admission criteria were predictive of which

> All admission criteria must be fair and reliable.

students will be successful. The expectation is that students who score well on admission criteria will score well in the nursing courses. Those scoring low on admission criteria would likely not perform as well in the nursing courses as those who scored higher. If the results indicate otherwise, then the admission criteria should be reconsidered.

PRINCIPLE

#14 New learning can only be based on what students have already learned.

The previous discussion on admission criteria relates to this Principle. A good part of my consulting business focuses on improving program completion rates. Many students struggle with the first term nursing courses. There are a number of reasons why successful completion of the first nursing courses is an issue, but I have discovered that one reason is because the courses taught in the first term require students to have knowledge beyond what was learned in the pre-requisite courses. For example, in a two-year nursing program, students may be asked to take the first course of a two-course sequence of anatomy and physiology as a pre-requisite to entering the program. The second course in the two-course sequence of anatomy and physiology is scheduled to be taken in the first term of the nursing program along with nursing courses. However, information taught in the first term nursing courses requires an understanding of the content of **both** anatomy and physiology courses, although only one was required prior to entering the nursing program. Some students did complete both courses and those students performed well in the nursing courses.

Other students who did not complete both anatomy and physiology courses struggled. Faculty may conclude that the admission criteria are not reliable or the students are not ready to enter the nursing program. Both these conclusions may be false. The real issue may be that students were not ready for the nursing courses because they did not complete the two anatomy and physiology courses. They were expected to apply content they had not yet learned.

> Plan course content and learning expectations that align with the curriculum.

This is a common example of not using the Principle: New learning can only be based on what students have already learned.

Faculty are responsible for planning course content and learning expectations that align with the curriculum. For this reason, all faculty must be very familiar with what is taught where in the nursing program to align course content based on the students' educational preparation.

PRINCIPLE
#15 Do you have a weed-out course?

Students once asked me if there is a "weed-out" course in the nursing program. I was surprised with the question because at that point in my career I had not heard of a "weed-out" course. They explained a "weed-out" course is one that "weeds out" the lower performing students so when the class graduates most of the graduates will pass NCLEX and give the school the pass rates the program needs to continue operating.

A variation of a "weed-out" course is a "weed-out" exam. A weed-out exam is the administration of a standardized comprehensive final exam with the requirement a student must earn a specific score. Student progression and graduation can be delayed or even prevented depending on the standardized exam score even if the student has passed all other course and program requirements.

It was easy to see that a "weed-out" course is a bad idea. But if a "weed-out" course is a bad idea would that same thinking apply to a required score on a standardized exam? If students have passed all course and program requirements why should their graduation be delayed because of a score on a standardized exam?

Nursing programs must set a high bar, but nursing programs must make getting over that bar doable. Education is expensive for students in terms of both time and dollars. Neither should be wasted.

> Nursing programs
> must set a high bar,
> but nursing programs
> must make getting over
> that bar doable.

PRINCIPLE

#16 Teach students that technology is important, but never more important than the patient.

There is an Indian proverb that states: A healthy person has lots of wishes; a sick person has just one. I truly think this proverb can be used to inspire nursing students to be empathetic and focused on the patient. When caring for the sick, the patient needs to receive care from a caring, focused, engaged nurse—as well as all other healthcare professionals!

I recently heard a nurse complain about a patient because the patient was upset the nurse was asking questions while focused on the computer screen and not making eye contact with the patient. The nurse complained the patient did not understand the importance of computer technology to provide safe patient care. As I'm listening to this nurse, I immediately thought, "Of course the patient didn't realize that!" The patient has but one wish—to get well and expects all healthcare providers to focus on that goal. A better approach for the nurse would have been to spend a couple of minutes looking directly at the patient (not the computer screen) and ask the patient how they are doing. After showing interest and concern, inform the patient the nurse will be asking more questions but will be looking at the computer to ensure their answers are entered correctly. Then when finished, once again look at the patient and once again engage directly with the patient showing empathy and concern.

When technology first appeared on the healthcare scene, nursing organizations adopted the slogan, "High tech, high touch." With the focus on technology and informatics, we must not forget the high touch.

> A healthy person
> has lots of wishes;
> a sick person
> has just one.

PRINCIPLE

#17 Fewer than 10% of new graduates demonstrate entry-level competence for clinical judgment in practice (Kavanagh & Sharpnack, 2021).

Nurse educators must be change agents—we must change not only the way we teach nursing students but also the way we teach nurse educators. To address the problem identified by Kavanagh and Sharpnack in 2021 (and a number of other studies prior to that 2021 manuscript), we must consider graduate level nursing education and how we are educating nursing educators. We need to change the curriculum in Masters, DNP, EdD, and PhD programs preparing academic nurse educators so the curriculum includes courses on how to teach students to think. The curriculum must include content about new, innovative ways to accomplish this task. What is currently being taught in these graduate programs is based on the decades old approach of "ask a lot of questions," "ask high cognitive level questions," and "use Socratic questioning." **This does not teach students to think; it requires students to use thinking they were never taught.**

As noted, research demonstrates new graduates are not able to think at safe levels which confirms the decades-old approach to teaching thinking does not work.

Some changes to consider include:

1. In the fundamentals course, immerse students in learning a clinical judgment framework that involves a very detailed, organized, structured way to think that will be used across the entire nursing program by all faculty.

2. All faculty use the clinical judgment framework as they direct student thinking in all educational settings including the clinical setting and simulation debriefing.

3. As discussed in previous Principles, revise homework assignments—the old "read and be prepared" is no longer appropriate. Completing pre-class worksheets focused on important information that students will use in the classroom when applying the clinical judgment framework is a change that can produce very positive outcomes (Bernard, Rosales, & Zurcher, 2022).

4. Include a graduate level course on how to teach nursing students to think. I hold a Masters in Nursing Education and a Doctorate in Education. I have taught in several masters in nursing education programs. None of these programs included a specific course on, or even included instruction about, how to teach students to think in a very detailed manner.

These are just some areas of change to consider—there are so many more! We must teach clinical judgment in a different way than what we have been doing for over 40 years—because that old way does not work.

We need to change the curriculum in Masters, DNP, EdD, and PhD programs preparing academic nurse educators so the curriculum includes courses on how to teach students to think.

PRINCIPLE

#18 Students should graduate from a pre-licensure nursing program as self-directed thinkers.

"Self-directed thinkers are independent thinkers who can explain their thinking, determine what thinking needs to be employed in a particular situation, then apply their thinking to arrive at a sound decision" (Caputi, 2022, p. 13).

The Next Generation NCLEX requires candidates to be self-directed thinkers. Candidates must be able to guide their own thinking to recognize what data are important, organize data, analyze data, and use that data to make well-informed decisions for safe patient care. This guidance of thinking is not based on content, such as, "What do I remember about postpartum care?" The student's thinking should apply clinical judgment competencies such as "Determining important information to collect" or "Judging how much ambiguity is acceptable." Using these and other clinical judgment competencies leads the student to the postpartum care nursing content needed for that particular patient. The thinking is guided by using thinking skills or clinical judgment competencies to direct thinking. Therefore, the nursing content the student needs to use is identified by applying the clinical judgment competencies. Without learning clinical judgment competencies, the student cannot learn to think. The thinking they do is based solely on recalling information, not on applying thinking.

> "Self-directed thinkers are independent thinkers who can explain their thinking, determine what thinking needs to be employed in a particular situation, then apply their thinking to arrive at a sound decision" (Caputi, 2022, p. 13).

Students must learn a detailed clinical judgment framework to become self-directed thinkers.

PRINCIPLE

#19 It's not the content that is tested, it's how the nurse uses the content.

This Principle is the message that was delivered by the National Council of State Boards of Nursing during the 2022 NCLEX conference. Of course, students learn content, but the NCLEX will test how they **use** the content in a patient situation. That type of testing is needed because nurses do not simply recall nursing information, but they use the information as they process and analyze patient information to plan safe patient care. Thus, the need for teaching and assessing students at the applying and higher cognitive levels.

Focus on **using content**, not on **memorizing** content. The more students use content by applying clinical judgment to individual patient care issues, the deeper

> Applying clinical judgment to content solidifies the content being learned.

the learning of that content will become. Applying clinical judgment to content solidifies the content being learned.

Other Principles in this section discuss specifics about teaching clinical judgment.

PRINCIPLE

#20 Teaching clinical judgment is so important because it is used in all nursing situations.

Like all fundamental concepts, clinical judgment cuts across all areas of nursing practice.

Ever have the experience of a student submitting a care plan after caring for a patient in the clinical and the care plan in no way relates to the individual patient the student cared for? The student used the course textbooks to determine how to care for a patient with a specific disease process, then copied information from the book without individualizing the information for the patient's unique situation. As a nursing faculty, this was my experience with such frequency that I had a stamp made that said, "Individualize for this patient." When grading handwritten care plans, I could merely stamp the paper rather than write that phrase over and over. It saved a lot of time and writing. However, just having to do this provided evidence that the current way of teaching care planning was not working! Students were not independent thinkers who could apply content to a specific patient situation through the use of clinical judgment.

Enter clinical judgment. Clinical judgment is the bridge that connects content learned in the classroom to nursing practice. Without clinical judgment students learn content but do not know how to apply that content during patient care or when dealing with other non-patient care nursing situations on a clinical unit. Rather than determine what to do by recalling previously learned information, students use clinical judgment competencies to determine what content to use then apply that content to a new, individual patient context. The same content may be used for two different patients with similar healthcare needs and disease processes. But how that content is applied to the two different patients is determined within the individual patient context. To work through the individual context for each patient, clinical judgment must be used.

> Clinical judgment is the bridge that connects nursing content and context that results in individualized patient care.

PRINCIPLE

#21 Clinical judgment is the overarching concept in all nursing programs at all levels of nursing practice.

Teaching clinical judgment should be the overarching concept in all nursing programs at all levels. To that end, it is extremely important to write a **specific** end-of-program learning outcome focused on clinical judgment because the research over the last 10 years demonstrates new nursing graduates are not thinking at the level needed for safe practice. The NCLEX changed starting April 1, 2023, to test clinical judgment because quality patient outcomes require the new graduate to be able to think. Writing a program learning outcome puts focus on clinical judgment as it does for any major concept that is the center of a program learning outcome such as safety, professionalism, and quality improvement. I recommend including a program learning outcome that specifically mentions the student using clinical judgment to elevate that concept to the level of other main concepts as written in the program learning outcomes. Here is an example end-of-program learning outcome focused on clinical judgment with related competencies.

Engage in clinical judgment when making patient-centered care and other nursing decisions.

1. Apply a clinical judgment framework to guide nursing practice.

2. Use clinical judgment competencies to ensure accurate and safe nursing care for the goal of improving patient outcomes.

3. Anticipate risks, and predict and manage potential complications.

4. Prioritize care based on individual patient/population needs.

As previously cited, the research on the thinking abilities of newly licensed Registered Nurses is dismal, in fact some call it a crisis (Kavanagh & Szweda, 2017). The latest research in 2021 indicated that less than 10% of newly licensed RNs can think at entry level expectations regardless of level of preparation (ASN, Diploma, or BSN) (Kavanagh & Sharpnack, 2021).

Nurse educators often state that students learn clinical judgment and problem solving in nursing by learning and using the nursing process. The issue with using the nursing process is that framework only provides general categories of thinking that need to be completed in the form of five steps. The nursing process does not teach the detailed thinking required for each of the five steps. The general nature of the nursing process is not enough to teach clinical judgment. This point was made by the NCSBN at the September, 2022, NCLEX workshop. It is critical students learn about the nursing process, but not as a detailed framework for thinking. The specific, detailed thinking of each of the five steps must be taught.

Clinical judgment is a hugely important concept that must be intentionally taught and learned in the first term of a nursing program, then applied across all nursing courses. The research on new graduates' ability to engage in clinical judgment indicates the current ways to teach clinical judgment are not working. It makes sense that the way we teach clinical judgment **must change**.

So, (1) what is the actual problem with the way we teach clinical judgment and (2) how can we change?

The actual problem is that clinical judgment itself is not actually taught. The NCSBN's clinical judgment measurement model (CJMM) is often used by many who purport to provide a new approach to teaching thinking. However, the purported new approach is the same approach to teaching thinking based on using the nursing process, but with new labels. The "new" approach now uses six general statements representing the six cognitive processes of the CJMM rather than the five steps of the nursing process. But the new process still does not teach the **detailed thinking** needed for an in-depth study of what clinical judgment is all about. In fact, the developers of the CJMM stress this is a **measurement model** and not a **teaching model**. The CJMM is intended for high-stakes testing (NCLEX) to measure the candidate's ability to use clinical judgment, and not for teaching (Dickison, Haerling, & Lasater, 2020).

The Next Generation NCLEX directly measures clinical judgment because new graduates are expected to learn and use clinical judgment. The NCSBN suggests that nursing programs teach a **framework** for clinical judgment. Using a framework is often suggested in the general nursing education literature as well. For example, Poledna, Gomez-Morales, and Hager (2022) studied students' use of thinking in simulation. They found students were not able to recognize cues indicating a change in the patient's condition. They noted that implementing a clinical judgment framework into the already existing nursing curriculum is a sound first step for developing cue recognition. Remember, cue recognition is just one of six cognitive processes tested on the Next Generation NCLEX. Thus, the need for an intense focus on teaching clinical judgment by using a very organized, detailed framework.

Teaching a detailed approach to clinical judgment is critically important so students actually learn about the concept of clinical judgment. Faculty must make a decision about what framework to use—should you use a general framework or a detailed framework? In addition to the nursing process, some nursing programs use Tanner's Clinical Judgment Model (2006). Tanner's model has just four very broad steps: (1) noticing, (2) interpreting, (3) responding, and (4) reflecting. What is sorely lacking are the specific thinking skills or clinical judgment competencies used in each of these four steps. The Tanner model does not drill down to the detailed thinking that is needed, but rather only addresses the four general steps. Dr. Tanner's work was seminal because it provided a different perspective on thinking than the nursing process. It was first published in 2006 and remains unchanged. It is the opinion of this author that the excellent work of Dr. Tanner needs to be updated and detailed, which is what the Caputi Clinical Judgment Framework has accomplished as discussed later in this Principle.

Traditionally, nursing educators expected students to use clinical judgment (the old term was critical thinking), but never actually taught clinical judgment. This is the same approach still used by many third-party resources claiming to teach clinical judgment. That approach wraps the old way in the new language of the NCSBN's CJMM. For example, some of these resources advise nursing programs to ask students questions that are arbitrarily aligned with one of the six clinical judgment cognitive processes of the NCSBN's clinical judgment measurement model. If students answer correctly, then the vendor says students are showing they can use clinical judgment. In reality, the only conclusion faculty can draw from a correct answer is that the student answered the question correctly. There is no evidence that the thinking of clinical judgment was used. Even asking students their "rationale" for their answer only requires students to explain content they used to answer the question such as lab results, symptoms of a disease process, or vital signs. It does not tell faculty anything about the thinking processes the student actually used to determine what content to use to formulate their answers.

As previously cited, faculty must realize the NCSBN's CJMM is intended for high-stakes testing and measurement on the NCLEX. It was not developed for teaching purposes. As advised by the developers of the model, nursing programs should carefully review clinical judgment models/frameworks and determine what is the best fit for their nursing program (Dickison, Haerling, Lasater, 2020).

To review: The old way of teaching thinking: Give students lots of case studies and ask lots of "clinical judgment" questions that are now aligned to one of the 6 cognitive processes of the NCSBN's CJMM. That approach **does not teach** clinical judgment. That process expects the students **to use** clinical judgment they have never actually learned.

So, what do you do?

Information shared by the NCSBN in the September, 2022, NCLEX conference stated the nursing process is not enough to teach thinking and a clinical judgment framework or model should be used. When deciding on a framework, consider the actual thinking processes nurses use. What are the thinking skills and strategies or clinical judgment competencies used in each step of the nursing process? This is the BIG missing piece. Faculty must drill down to the detailed thinking and walk students step-by-step through that thinking as they learn each clinical judgment competency. This detailed framework is taught in the first term of a nursing program, then ALL faculty use that same framework as they engage students in clinical judgment throughout the entire program. This is the only way to get to the detail of what needs to be taught to learn clinical judgment and to develop self-directed thinkers by completion of the program.

Teaching a Clinical Judgment Framework

The following explains an approach to teaching clinical judgment I developed and have used throughout the last 15 years with over 250 schools. I am sharing in this Principle information about the current version of my approach. I am sharing this information because there is no other source that provides information about how to **actually teach the clinical judgment process**.

Clinical judgment in nursing needs to be taught in the first term of nursing in a separate course—or if this isn't possible—deliberately integrated into the first clinical course. A separate course is the ideal approach because it decreases the risk of the clinical judgment content getting lost in a course, something that occasionally happens when content is "integrated" into another course.

Teaching a clinical judgment framework (Tyo & McCurry, 2019) is the best approach because it breaks down clinical judgment into its component parts including individual thinking skills and strategies (clinical judgment competencies). Once taught in the first term, the thinking skills and the framework in which they reside, must be emphasized and applied to nursing practice in all other nursing courses and in all teaching/learning environments (classroom, laboratory, and clinical) across the program. Throughout the initial teaching of clinical judgment and application across the nursing program, faculty design learning activities to deliberately engage students as they use each of the clinical judgment competencies in the classroom, simulation debriefing, and clinical.

In a course in the first term of the nursing program, break down clinical judgment into its component thinking skills (clinical judgment competencies). These clinical judgment competencies are then used and built on throughout the program in the classroom, simulation, and clinical. Without providing a specific focus on thinking at applying and higher levels in your program, students will not be prepared for the Next Gen NCLEX.

Remember: The Next Gen NCLEX-RN and NCLEX-PN both include clinical judgment as an integrated concept—in the same manner as spirituality, the nursing process, caring, and the other integrated processes. An integrated process is one that is fundamental to the practice of nursing and integrated throughout the Client Needs categories and subcategories on the detailed NCLEX test plans (NCSBN, 2023). As an integrated concept, clinical judgment type of thinking can be required when answering all test items not just the questions in the Next Gen NCLEX formats.

The framework I developed for teaching clinical judgment and clinical judgment competencies is in the student textbook *Think Like a Nurse: The Caputi Method for Learning Clinical Judgment*. It is the only nursing student textbook that actually teaches students a thinking process that covers all the thinking skills, how to use them, and how to use them as a framework when faced with new situations that require clinical judgment. The below table aligns the cognitive processes of the NCSBN's Clinical Judgment Measurement Model to my five-step framework with examples of the **detailed** clinical judgment competencies (thinking skills and strategies) needed to implement each of the NCSBN's cognitive processes.

Note: The Cognitive Processes of the NCSBN's Clinical Judgment Measurement Model are noted in parentheses and bolded. NP means Nursing Process.

Major Steps in the Caputi Clinical Judgment Framework	The Caputi Clinical Judgment (CJ) Competencies
1. Getting the Information (Recognize Cues) NP: Assessing	1. Determining important information to collect 2. Scanning the environment 3. Identifying signs and symptoms *There are 2 more CJ competencies.*
2. Making Meaning of the Information (Analyze Cues) NP: Diagnosing: Identifying Patient Problems	1. Clustering related information 2. Identifying assumptions 3. Recognizing inconsistencies 4. Distinguishing relevant from irrelevant information 5. Judging how much ambiguity is acceptable *There are 4 more CJ competencies.*
3. Determining Actions to Take (Prioritize Hypotheses and Generate Solutions) NP: Planning	1. Selecting interventions 2. Managing potential complications 3. Setting priorities
4. Taking Action (Take Actions) NP: Implementing	1. Determining how to implement the planned interventions 2. Delegating *There are 2 more CJ competencies.*
5. Evaluating Outcomes and Your Thinking (Evaluate Outcomes) NP: Evaluating	1. Evaluating data 2. Evaluating and correcting thinking

The Caputi Clinical Judgment Framework drills down to the specific clinical judgment competencies students must learn in preparation for taking the Next Generation NCLEX. For more information please visit: https://lindacaputi.com/about-the-book/.

To reiterate, it is critical to teach clinical judgment by using a framework such as the one presented in this Principle. This is a common theme throughout the clinical judgment research.

All nursing programs must place a much stronger emphasis on teaching the clinical judgment process both for the Next Generation NCLEX and for preparation for safe practice. Clinical judgment must be learned to support the thinking that is used when applying the nursing process. Graduate programs that prepare academic nurse educators should consider developing a course that teaches faculty how to teach nursing students to think. If faculty do not learn this process, how will they know how to teach their students clinical judgment? Clinical judgment is the most important concept to teach in all nursing programs at all levels of nursing.

> All nursing programs must place a much stronger emphasis on teaching the clinical judgment process, both for the Next Generation NCLEX and for preparation for safe practice.

PRINCIPLE

#22 Replace 5-column care plans with concept maps.

I am often asked the question: "Care plans versus concept maps, which is better?" Concept maps used to replace traditional care plans are often called care maps. When considering the "why" for assigning care plans, ask: "What is the goal you are trying to achieve by assigning a 5-column care plan?" The goal might be to determine if students can fill in the five columns with information typical of a care plan. However, the overarching lesson should be that the student can demonstrate knowledge of the five steps of the nursing process using clinical judgment applied to a specific patient situation. It actually took me 20 years of grading care plans and writing over and over, "Individualize for this patient" before I realized this assignment did not provide evidence of achieving its intended purpose. Perhaps it is time for a change.

The typical undergraduate care plan assignment consists of a rather lengthy (sometimes as many as 35 pages) "fill-in-the-blank" assessment completed while in the clinical setting. The 5-column care plan itself is then completed either in clinical, or, more commonly, outside of the clinical setting. Students use the information from the lengthy assessment as the basis for identifying patient issues, problems, concerns (diagnoses). Nursing interventions are then listed for the care required for the identified patient issues. The final column is used to record evaluation data and changes that should be made based on collected evaluation data.

Students often complete the 5-column care plan by copying information from a textbook, care plan book, nursing diagnosis book, or some other source. This is evident because the plan of care often is not individualized to the patient.

Another issue with the care plan assignment is it represents the end product of thinking. It may or may not be the student's thinking. There is also no indication of the student's thinking that led to the information placed on the care plan. There is no direct connection of the student's thinking to the entries on the care plan.

Is this the case with concept maps? The purpose of concept maps is to provide a window into the student's mind, into the way the student is thinking. True concept maps actually do provide that information. However, to understand the student's thinking when constructing the concept map, there are some factors about concept maps faculty should consider.

1. A concept map is a diagram that represents the relationship between and among concepts or ideas. A concept map is also called a mind map because it reflects the thinking of the developer. The student uses geometric figures to contain the information with lines to connect the geometric figures. The student notes on each line one or two words that indicate how the two concepts link together. Each concept may have connecting lines from one or more concepts as needed.

2. Concept maps are valuable because the student creates them based on their own thinking. Students should start with a blank piece of paper then add concepts and lines as they work through the assignment. They should not be directed what information to enter where. That is, the geometric figures should not be prelabeled with words such as those of the five steps of the nursing process. When this type of prelabeled map is used, the student is putting the information that would be placed in a 5-column care plan into the geometric figures. Students are not making their own connections, rather the faculty is making the connections for them. The student is merely filling in the information based on the labels.

3. Concept maps should unfold as the student applies thinking when engaging in the activity or with the material. Students should use the detailed clinical judgment framework that provides specific clinical judgment competencies (thinking skills). Applying those thinking skills leads the student to the information to be placed on the concept map. This process reflects reality because this is what nurses do—nurses use thinking to determine what information to collect, to make meaning of the information they collect, then to determine what to do. For most nurses, this is an intuitive process and they are unaware of the thinking that is occurring. For students this is **not** an intuitive process so they must have cognitive guidance to determine how to think.

4. When replacing care plans in the clinical with concept maps the student should start at the beginning of the clinical time with a blank piece of paper. Some patient information from report can be inserted into a circle in the middle of the paper. The student then uses the clinical judgment competencies to guide their thinking.

5. For example, the patient's temperature is 101.8. The student draws a line from the middle circle to a square. On the line the student writes "Determining important information to collect" and in the square writes: T-101.8. This demonstrates the student used the clinical judgment competency to decide what information is important. So, how would the nurse think about this temperature? The nurse would determine what other information is important to consider for the elevated temperature. The student draws a line off the temperature square and on that line writes: "Assessing systematically and comprehensively." Then draws a rectangle. In that rectangle the student writes other information to collect to ensure a comprehensive assessment related to the elevated temperature is performed. The student writes information such as: "check WBCs" then inserts information into a figure with the results of the WBCs; "trend previous WBC results" and includes those in the rectangle; "Check MAR" and writes in any antipyretic or antimicrobials ordered. This continues as the student connects previously learned information useful to the findings for the patient with a fever. Of course, the concept map continues to unfold as the student adds lines labeled with other clinical judgment competencies and the information yielded as a result of using those competencies.

6. A concept map can become full of information with lots of connecting lines. For this reason, the student must verbally explain the entries and lines as the concept map is unfolding across the clinical day. It will be difficult for faculty to clearly understand all the entries and their connections without the student's explanations.

7. As students explain their entries on the concept map, faculty can assess the student's ability to engage in thinking.

8. For clinical concept maps that replace care plans, the concept map unfolds and builds across the clinical day. Faculty interact frequently with students as they explain how their map is unfolding. For this reason, the unfolding concept map is written while in the clinical setting. Faculty provide ongoing feedback across the clinical day so the concept maps are graded while in clinical.

The concept map and implementation of the concept map assignment explained above renders the concept map superior to the 5-column care plan even if the 5-column care plan is completed during clinical time. The traditional 5-column care plan does not provide any evidence of the student's ability to engage in clinical judgment and that is a critical reason to use the concept map activity.

It actually took me 20 years
of grading care plans and
writing over and over,
"Individualize for this
patient" before I realized this
assignment did not provide
evidence of achieving its
intended purpose.

Perhaps it is time for a change.

PRINCIPLE

#23 Saying "It's just common sense" does not make sense to new learners.

Students occasionally report to faculty that when they asked a nurse a question about why the nurse was doing what they were doing, the nurse would often respond, "It's just common sense." Because expert nurses no longer think about rationales and explanations, but operate from a deep understanding of nursing applied to complex, varied, and plentiful patient experiences, so much of what is done just seems to be common sense. It is understandable that expert nurses would answer in this manner.

However, the commonsense answer by faculty is not helpful to students. Although nursing faculty have typically reached an expert level of functioning with much of what they do based on intuition (which appears to be common sense), faculty must be able to articulate the thinking they used (clinical judgment), explain rationales, and provide in-depth explanations. Nursing care only becomes "common sense" once the nurse has a deep understanding of, and multiple experiences in, nursing.

Nurses are not able to achieve a "common sense" level of functioning until they become experts in their practice.

> Nursing care only becomes
> "common sense" once
> the nurse has a deep
> understanding of, and multiple
> experiences in, nursing.

PRINCIPLE
#24   We need not be afraid to question and reconsider.

As I work, consider, apply, analyze, and evaluate an intense focus on teaching clinical judgment in nursing programs, I wonder if anyone would be so brave as to question Dr. Benner's Novice to Expert theory. The Novice to Expert theory has lived in nursing since the middle 1980s. As Dr. Benner did her work measuring how nurses acquire skill in thinking, the subjects of her research were all taught to think in the way that was customary in those years. Teaching thinking in those years (and still is today) did not actually teach thinking itself, but was all about asking students lots of probing questions and using Socratic questioning to foster "critical thinking" as it was called during that time.

Consider a paradigm shift in nursing education that teaches clinical judgment differently. Students initially learn a systematic, formalized, deliberate framework with specific clinical judgment competencies (Caputi, 2022). Students then use that framework across the nursing program curriculum to emerge as self-directed thinkers by graduation. Would this higher level of thinking by new graduates change the trajectory through the five steps of the Novice to Expert theory? Can a change in the way we teach thinking (clinical judgment) affect the findings of a study that replicates Dr. Benner's research?

> Can a change in the way we teach clinical judgment influence a student's trajectory from Novice to Expert?

Shall we ask the question: "What outcome will teaching clinical judgment in a formalized, systematic, detailed way have on a nurse's path from Novice to Expert?"

PRINCIPLE

#25 All faculty in pre-licensure nursing programs are NCLEX coaches.

There is no need for a separate NCLEX coach or for a standardized testing company to be in charge of the task of preparing your students for NCLEX. Beginning in the middle 1990s nursing faculty have been told by a number of entities that they are not NCLEX experts—that they need help from an outside source that "specializes" in preparing students for NCLEX. Many faculty have come to believe that messaging.

There is nothing magical about NCLEX that all faculty cannot learn about and prepare students for that exam. In fact, in a pre-licensure nursing program, it is the **faculty's responsibility** to prepare students for the NCLEX. Information about NCLEX is available to everyone at the NCSBN.com website and other NCSBN supported websites such as NextGenNurses.org and NCLEX.com. All faculty have access to this information. It is the same information that NCLEX preparation companies and standardized testing companies access. Everyone has access to the same information so everyone is able to learn about the NCLEX.

I often find nursing programs put the teaching of nursing into one silo and preparation for NCLEX in another silo. Contents of the silos are as follows:

Teaching Nursing Silo #1: All the curriculum components of the program: the course syllabi, required textbooks, reading assignments for the courses, exams focused on the course content, etc.

NCLEX Preparation Silo #2: (a) NCLEX related materials typically supplied by a third-party NCLEX preparation vendor including nursing content books, online activities, practice exams, remediation materials, proctored testing, etc., (b) An "NCLEX coach" or adviser position who oversees the standardized assignments and testing, making sure it is all in place; provides students NCLEX coaching in some format that is separate from the nursing program curriculum.

These approaches to curriculum and NCLEX preparation should not be separate entities. It is best for **all** faculty to:

1. Be an NCLEX expert keeping current about what is happening with NCLEX by studying the NCSBN.org website and the other two websites from the NCSBN cited earlier. Teaching for success on NCLEX involves teaching content (#2 below) and teaching clinical judgment (#3 below). Faculty must address both.

2. Use the **detailed NCLEX test plan** every day in all learning environments—but especially in the theory classroom. Require students to actively use the test plan in class. See the "how to" section following this list.

3. Teach a detailed clinical judgment framework to prepare students for the Next Gen NCLEX.

4. Eliminate the second curriculum represented in Silo #2 and ensure the program's curriculum covers what is needed for success on the NCLEX. Students often complain they are required to learn two curricula and the two curricula do not match.

5. Write items for classroom practice and teacher-made exams that are in the form used on NCLEX. Faculty become knowledgeable about how to categorize the cognitive level of test items according to each level of Bloom's taxonomy. This means accurately identifying the type of thinking the student must use to answer each of the test items and aligning that thinking to the correct level on the taxonomy. As previously noted, faculty often hear that they are not "testing experts, so leave the testing to the experts." Nothing could be further from the truth! It is the faculty's responsibility to learn to write solid test items that test content AND clinical judgment. You can do it; don't let anyone tell you that you cannot!

6. Provide faculty-mediated remediation so all students are provided the guidance needed to answer test items, but more importantly to "fill in the gaps" of content and thinking.

7. Involve students in their study and planning for NCLEX. Use a tool such as the *Student Self-Checklist for NCLEX Success* included in the Appendices of this book. Faculty may use this tool as is or revise it for their specific student needs.

How To Use the Detailed NCLEX Test Plan in the Classroom

In this section I am sharing an approach I have been using with schools for over 15 years. It has been very successful as one aspect of NCLEX preparation.

This intervention requires students to use the **detailed NCLEX test plan** in class every day so students become totally familiar with, and use, the detailed test plan throughout the nursing program. **It is the student who will be taking NCLEX** so it is critical the student thoroughly learns and uses the detailed test plan.

1. Provide students with a hard copy of the **detailed NCLEX** test plan. On that hard copy, number each of the detailed objectives. Of course, the ones in the boxes at the beginning of each major category are repeated throughout that section so you do not need to number the ones in the box.

2. Students bring the numbered print version of the test plan with them to class each day. For the last 15 minutes of each classroom session divide the students into groups with each group focusing on one of the eight major areas of NCLEX.

3. Ask each group to put the day's date next to each of the detailed objectives that relates to the class discussion that day. **It is critical that students are the ones who connect the detailed objectives to what was taught in class.** It does not help for faculty to read off the numbers of what they will be covering in class without students doing this active work.

4. Each group then shares the numbers next to the items they decided were addressed in class and all students make the date notation next to the objectives as indicated by the group reporting their findings.

5. The next day in class each group is assigned to a different category on the NCLEX test plan as the groups rotate through the major categories. This process provides students with lots of experience reviewing and making meaning out of the many

detailed objectives on the NCLEX test plan. They become very familiar with what is expected of them on the NCLEX. An added bonus is that students immediately review everything that was discussed in class helping them to solidify the day's learning.

In preparation for class, faculty should review the entire detailed test plan and put the date next to the objectives that will be covered that day. When students read the numbers of the objectives they selected, faculty can ensure they already identified them, and if not, faculty can add the date to their copy. Faculty can also inform students of any objectives the students missed.

Completing this exercise throughout the entire nursing program familiarizes students with the detailed NCLEX test plan. If they are having difficulty with an area, they can go back to that day's notes to review. Faculty can track any objectives not dated to see what is missing in your program.

Finally, student confidence in taking the NCLEX is heightened because they know from this tracking that everything on the NCLEX has been covered during the nursing program. Of course, the challenges are to: (1) address all these detailed objectives many times in the program, and (2) not just teach the content but engage students in activities using that content by applying higher levels of thinking requiring the use of clinical judgment. Then you test to all those detailed objectives, or in some way evaluate student learning related to the detailed objectives.

But Isn't This "Teaching to the Test?"

The phrase "teaching to the test" refers to faculty addressing **specific content** that will be covered on an exam. No one but the NCSBN knows exactly what specific content will be on the NCLEX. Let's take a deeper dive at what this means.

For classroom teaching, faculty prepare lesson objectives. These are shared with students. Here are example lesson objectives for an Adult Health class session:

1. Analyze patient situations to plan patient-centered care.

2. Determine potential problems related to elimination for select renal diseases.

3. Determine which interrelated concepts are important in planning care for two patients with renal disease.

4. Provide a safe environment for patients with issues with elimination.

5. When discussing nursing care identify other members of the healthcare team to consult.

Faculty share with students the above lesson objectives as they teach content that aligns with each objective. These lesson objectives do not indicate the exact content that will be on an exam. Rather, these learning objectives guide the students' learning and study for the exam. For example, there will be questions on the exam that require students to "Determine potential problems related to elimination for select renal diseases." The educator is not "teaching to the test" by providing these lesson objectives.

Now let's look at examples of detailed objectives on the NCLEX-RN:

1. Assess client care area for sources of infection.

2. Understand communicable diseases and the modes of organism transmission (e.g., airborne, droplet, contact).

3. Apply principles of infection prevention (e.g., hand hygiene, aseptic technique, isolation, sterile technique, universal/ standard enhanced barrier precautions).

When students connect the information presented in class to these NCLEX-RN detailed objectives, they are learning to identify information that represents these objectives and practice using information related to these objectives. However, they are not learning what specific content will be on the NCLEX nor how the questions will be asked. In fact, no one but the National Council of State Boards of Nursing knows exactly what content is on the exam.

For this reason, using the detailed NCLEX test plans in this manner is **NOT** teaching to the test because faculty do not know what content will be on the exam. All that is known by way of the NCLEX detailed test plans are the general detailed objectives. It is the faculty's responsibility to teach course content that aligns with these general objectives.

This Principle is extremely important for faculty who teach in pre-licensure nursing programs. As addressed in Chapter 1: Who You Are as Nurse Educator, you have or are developing your self-concept as a teacher of nursing. If you teach in a pre-licensure nursing program it is important to incorporate the responsibility of preparing students for NCLEX as part of your self-concept as a teacher. It is not an outside company's responsibility, but the responsibility of every faculty to prepare their students for NCLEX.

There is no need for a separate NCLEX coach or for a standardized testing company to be in charge of the task of preparing your students for NCLEX.

PRINCIPLE

#26
Provide an intense, in-house NCLEX preparation course focused on YOUR students' needs rather than use a canned, off-the-shelf review provided by an outside entity.

As previously stated, preparation for NCLEX requires students to learn both content and clinical judgment. Nursing programs should include in the last term of a nursing program a comprehensive course that provides a synthesis of all nursing concepts and content taught throughout the program with application of clinical judgment using case-based learning in the classroom. This course provides both individualized, and cohort focused, content review in preparation for the NCLEX rather than an "off-the-shelf" NCLEX review. An "off-the-shelf" NCLEX review may not address your individual student or cohort needs. A synthesis course enables the individual student to recognize areas that need enhancement prior to taking the NCLEX and entering nursing practice. The case-based learning approach requires faculty to use patient cases to apply the content using clinical judgment. Because both content and clinical judgment are measured on the NCLEX, teaching to both must be specifically planned. This course should also include a review of strategies for success on the NCLEX.

At the beginning of the final term, administer a comprehensive exam that provides direction about what content will be taught in the course. Here are two ways to determine what to include on that comprehensive exam:

1. All course faculty review the results of exams given in their courses to identify weak areas of performance. Include in the course these weak areas of content.

2. Refer to your program's most recent NCLEX Program Reports purchased from Mountain Measurement. Look at these for the lowest scoring content areas.

Once you have gathered the above information, construct an exam with questions from all content areas addressing the weak areas of performance. Faculty may use some previously administered questions, but revise them somewhat so the answers are different. This may be an easier way to construct the exam than writing totally new questions.

An alternative approach to the faculty constructed exam is to use a comprehensive exam from one of the standardized testing companies. The fear is those exams may be readily available for students to purchase on the internet. Just as textbook test banks have been available for years for students to purchase on the internet, so are the exams from standardized testing companies. This has been the case for a number of years and there is no reason to believe this will change. This problem of unauthorized distribution of these exams grew larger during the pandemic when exams were all taken remotely. However, this problem did not begin with the pandemic and it will not end with the end of the pandemic. If students have accessed these exams prior to taking the exam as part of a course, then the exam is NOT a reliable indicator of student learning. Faculty will be working with results that are not useful. For this reason, it is best for faculty to develop their own comprehensive exam based on what was taught across the program. However, if an exam purchased from a third-party vendor is used, this is the only time I recommend using a standardized exam in the nursing program.

The course starts with the administration of the comprehensive exam. Faculty examine the student results to determine the content areas with the weakest performance. The rest of the weeks in the course focus on the weak areas of student performance as a group as identified by the comprehensive exam, the weak areas of performance on classroom exams, and the low scoring areas on the Mountain Measurement Program Reports. Because the purpose of this course is to ensure all content related to the weak areas is taught, the course focuses specifically on areas of weakness.

The exam primarily provides information about weak areas of **content**. It does not provide information about weaknesses in clinical judgment. Therefore, the weekly class sessions should not be strictly lecture, but application of the content to complex patient care scenarios and case studies applying the clinical judgment framework students learned and applied throughout the program. Complex patient care scenarios do not refer to critical care patients, but to patients with multiple health problems.

During the course, faculty develop several classroom exams. These exams cover the content taught to the entire group.

Additionally, each student makes an individualized plan to study their own weak areas. These weak areas are determined by their individual performance on the comprehensive exam as well as content of nursing course with their lowest earned grades. Individual students may have weak areas that are not weak areas of the group. Including content from courses in which the student earned the lowest grades provides an additional individualized focus. Students must show evidence of studying these weak areas by completing a set number of NCLEX style questions on those topics and pass practice exams at a prescribed minimum level. These questions and practice exams can be taken from a number of sources. There are many sources of practice NCLEX items from various vendors. Search the ones that meet your needs that are the least expensive for your students.

A cumulative final exam covering all the content in the course is given at the end of the course. Faculty may also choose to administer a second comprehensive exam from an outside vendor. Use these results to:

1. Determine gains in learning achieved as a result of the course.

2. Use as a guide for students to develop an NCLEX preparation plan for their individual study after they graduate and prior to taking the NCLEX. Faculty work individually with each student to develop a study plan. This plan is for their own personal use.

At the end of the course when students receive their results from the cumulative final exam you develop and/or from the second comprehensive exam, they still only have feedback on content areas to study. Therefore, post-graduation study only involves content. The practice of applying clinical judgment must come during class time throughout the course to enhance and apply the clinical judgment framework students used across the program.

All faculty are NCLEX coaches; there is no need to delegate this role to an outside vendor. Also, nursing programs need an NCLEX preparation course that is focused on THEIR students' needs rather than a canned, off-the-shelf review course.

Creating an end-of-program faculty provided NCLEX review course that is totally focused on your students' needs is your gift to your graduating students.

PRINCIPLE

#27 A high NCLEX pass rate is desirable but not at the cost of a good completion rate.

Faculty often consider the NCLEX pass rate of another school and are amazed when it is 90% or higher. That level pass rate is very desirable. However, we must look at the total picture. What is the nursing program's completion rate? If only 50 or 60% of students complete the program, then the 90% or higher pass rate tends to lose its shine.

On the other hand, a nursing program may have a high completion rate but a low NCLEX pass rate. This may indicate grade inflation or nursing exams that are not at the cognitive level required to pass NCLEX. Students complete the program but do not do well on NCLEX.

Perhaps consider my mantra of 90/90. That is, aim for a 90% or higher completion rate and 90% or higher NCLEX pass rate and **believe** it can be done. It can be done, no matter the type of students in your nursing program. Learning about student characteristics and using those characteristics to guide delivery of the curriculum is key to success. Implement teaching and learning practices as discussed throughout this chapter. Consider all these practices and formulate a plan to realize a 90/90 outcome.

Faculty must strive for a high completion rate and a high NCLEX pass rate. Students deserve no less.

> Aim for a 90% or higher
> completion rate,
> and 90% or higher
> NCLEX pass rate,
> and believe it can be done.

PRINCIPLE
#28 KISS—Keep It Simple Scholar!

I agree with what the KISS acronym is saying in principle, but I do not accept the common interpretation of the acronym which is: Keep It Simple Stupid. It is not in my character to call others stupid. I prefer to interpret KISS as Keep It Simple Scholar.

Faculty are scholarly people who teach others. And teaching, simply put, is NOT just talking. Teaching requires faculty to apply learning strategies to turn content into something students can understand and use.

The KISS acronym should be applied to the teaching process. How can you turn what may be considered difficult content to understand into something that is meaningful and not difficult to learn? For example, using constructivist learning theory you help learners build on previous experiences and understandings to construct new and/or deeper understandings. This is sometimes referred to as expanding the students' cognitive frameworks—how they think about something.

I used constructivist learning theory in my student textbook *Think Like a Nurse: The Caputi Method for Learning Clinical Judgment*. For each clinical judgment competency, I:

1. First present how that thinking is used in everyday life and provide an everyday example.

2. Students then provide examples of how they use the clinical judgment competency in their everyday life.

3. Then I discuss how that same thinking—thinking students already know how to do—is applied to a simple nursing example.

4. Students then expand on their previous understanding of the clinical judgment competency (thinking skill) by using active learning in the classroom to apply that thinking to nursing.

This approach also empowers students because they realize they already know how to think, so they may already know something about clinical judgment. However, they have not actually considered the thinking processes they use when engaging in decision-making. They did not have the language to describe their thinking nor did they organize their thinking into a framework. They possibly did not realize they were even using thinking skills. Furthermore, as nursing students encounter new experiences, they continuously update their cognitive framework (mental model) as they use clinical judgment in more complex nursing situations.

This approach to teaching using constructivist learning theory provides a simple, understandable way to learn the complex concept of clinical judgment. We must make learning doable because **teaching only happens when learning takes place**.

We do not need to make learning nursing difficult—use KISS!

Teaching only happens
when learning takes place.

PRINCIPLE
#29 Always know the WHY behind the WHAT.

In the 1980s, a faculty colleague and I developed some of the first "computer-assisted instruction" software programs for nursing education. What an outdated term: "computer-assisted instruction!" That was, of course, before the internet. Terms such as "web-based instruction" replaced that old software term.

As we were developing these computer programs, we hired a graphic artist to develop very (at the time) sophisticated animations. One groundbreaking animation was a stick figure nurse pushing a wheelchair across the screen. Every time the student correctly answered a question, the nurse pushed the wheelchair a little closer to the Exit. Faculty and students using the program were so impressed! They loved seeing the nurse cross the screen as a visual indicator of their progress. We shared that response with the animator, and he said, "You always get them with the graphics!"

So, what's the problem with that thinking? The problem is this: Nothing in an educational program should be used unless it contributes to the students' learning. The time students spent watching the animated nurse push the patient in the wheelchair across the screen was a total waste. When I started my Doctor of Education program one of the first lessons I learned was, "Only use media if it contributes to the students' learning." The stick figure nurse pushing a wheelchair across the screen a number of times in that "tutorial" did NOT contribute to the students' learning. Some may say it motivated the students to do better because the nurse moved a short distance each time the student answered a question correctly. However, the motivation soon diminished and eventually the animation was more of an irritant than a motivator.

The lesson here is: Have a good reason for what you are using in your teaching/learning sessions and ensure what you use contributes to the students' learning. Clearly identify what learning you expect students to achieve. Clearly identify the cognitive level of thinking students need to use to complete the activity.

Here are some examples of when we should be questioning what we are doing:

1. If you play a Jeopardy or use other games in the classroom, why are you using the game? What is the purpose? Does it contribute to the students' learning? Is it a "drill and practice" activity used to engage students in recalling information as a form of review of content, but not application of content?

2. If you ask students to read 200 pages for next week's classroom session, why are they reading all 200 pages? What is the focus of the reading? What is the important content? What pages of the reading should students not read?

3. Never use technology just to use technology—every "medium" is used for an educational purpose to achieve an identified outcome. Always have an educational reason for using technology. Do not use technology (or any other medium) just to be using technology if there is not an educational reason for doing so.

Clearly identify the reasons for why you are doing what you are doing.

Nothing in an educational
program should be used
unless it contributes to the
students' learning.

PRINCIPLE
#30 Teach to current practice.

Teach to current practice when teaching content **and** thinking! Identify better ways to teach to make sure you are focused on current practice.

A perfect example of making a shift to teaching to current practice is clinical education. The old approach to teaching students in the clinical setting demonstrates the type of clinical environment that was present in the 1970s, 1980s, and early 1990s. Lots of things changed in the 1990s with Diagnosis Related Groups (DRGs) and changes in medical practice such as laparoscopic surgeries. Patients were no longer in the acute care setting for long periods of time "recovering"—many patients were not admitted but treated in out-patient healthcare agencies. Since that time, the clinical setting has continued to change and evolve in many different ways. Most patients who are admitted to an acute care setting are very ill or they would not be admitted.

Since that time, clinical education in pre-licensure nursing programs basically has not changed. The approach that continues through today involves:

1. Faculty make specific patient assignments for each student.
2. Some faculty require students to visit the healthcare agency to collect information and start a care plan the day before clinical.
3. The student works with the nurse to provide total care for the patient.
4. Students complete as many tasks as possible attempting to complete all tasks on time.
5. When students are not busy, they volunteer to help other nursing students, nurses, or nursing assistants.
6. Students collect patient information throughout the day then develop a care plan or concept map outside of clinical time.
7. Students submit the completed care plan to faculty to grade and provide feedback outside of clinical time.

The level of patient acuity is higher now than it has ever been. Nurses make many critical decisions each day, yet many schools continue to use this decades-old approach to teaching in the clinical setting that is primarily focused on completing tasks without any time devoted to using clinical judgment.

The critical piece that is missing in this decades-old approach is clinical judgment. What clinical judgment framework is used and how do students use that framework throughout the clinical day to think like a nurse? Can students take time in clinical to engage in clinical judgment rather than always engaging in tasks? If the nurse engages in thinking throughout the clinical day, shouldn't the student? To teach to current practice, we must ask: "How much time does a nurse spend thinking?" Then we must require students to engage in lots of time thinking **while in the clinical**.

> If the nurse engages in thinking throughout the clinical day, shouldn't the student?

Analyze current practice, determine what a nurse does and how a nurse infuses thinking throughout the day, then use that to guide your students' clinical experience.

PRINCIPLE

#31 What happens in clinical stays in clinical.

It is important to consider clinical homework and how much time students spend outside of clinical to complete the work. How much time do students spend writing care plans or completing other clinical-related homework? Do you have evidence the clinical homework enhances student learning?

I suggest students spend very little time outside of clinical completing clinical homework. Consider this: For every credit hour assigned to a clinical course, students typically are present in clinical for 3 clock hours. For a classroom course, students are in class 1 clock hour for every credit hour. This is because the classroom does not include homework time. Students must put in 3 clock hours of effort for every credit hour earned. Students are expected to complete 2 clock hours of study engaging in outside of class homework for every credit hour.

For clinical, students are putting in all 3 clock hours for each credit hour for learning and homework time while they are present in the clinical setting. To require students to spend many clock hours outside of clinical completing clinical assignments impinges on their out-of-class study time and is not necessary to complete the requirements to earn credit hours.

I suggest revising clinical assignments so students are assigned fewer patients but with a more in-depth study of that patient using different approaches rather than long care plans or pre-populated concept maps. Students should receive immediate feedback on these assignments. Use activities that require students to apply the clinical judgment framework to patient care. Students should be allowed to work on these assignments while in the clinical setting. This should not be taboo.

Students can complete the "care plan" in the clinical setting in a newly revised format. This new format breaks down all the pieces of the large care plan assignment and inserts thinking into the assignment based on the detailed clinical judgment framework learned. Students then complete the various pieces of the care plan throughout the clinical time. This approach combines patient care and clinical judgment. This is similar to the unfolding concept map previously discussed.

Application of clinical judgment is essential for current practice. Receiving and using feedback on clinical judgment activities needs to be an integral part of the clinical experience. Faculty can develop a grading rubric for each smaller assignment for easy grading and providing feedback to students while still in the clinical setting. This type of detailed, immediate feedback is more valuable and results in greater learning than grading care plans completed out of the clinical setting after the clinical day. By the time students receive the feedback they may no longer remember much of what they experienced. A basic educational principle is that the closer the feedback is to the learning behavior, the more effective the feedback is for student growth.

Remember: Learning to think like a nurse is not confined to the classroom on campus. Clinical judgment must be applied in the clinical setting. Student assignments should demonstrate application of content with deliberate use of clinical judgment when providing individualized patient care. Currently, there is very little application of clinical judgment in the clinical setting of educational programs (Nielsen, et al., 2023).

Faculty may need to talk with the clinical staff to inform them students are not "doing their homework" but "recording their thinking." Remember, staff were educated in the old way of clinical education that required them to collect all that information then spend long hours at home completing the work. They then submitted the work to faculty. The faculty (who are no longer in the clinical) grade the assignments and return the assignments to students long after the clinical day. Faculty may need to educate clinical staff on this new way of doing.

> Immediately receiving feedback on clinical judgment activities needs to be an integral part of the clinical experience.

A new way of teaching and learning in the clinical is sorely needed. The above approach operationalizes this Principle: What happens in clinical stays in clinical.

PRINCIPLE

#32 Thinking must occur in the clinical setting with as much time dedicated to thinking as doing.

Do not hesitate to try a new approach to teaching in the clinical setting. The approach discussed in Principle #31 in this chapter replaces the old "non-stop performing tasks" and keeping busy, with an approach that focuses on both hands-on care and clinical judgment. The new approach requires students to spend 50% of clinical time performing tasks and 50% focusing on thinking like a nurse. The approach of writing a very long care plan or filling in pre-labeled geometric figures on a concept map is the traditional way clinical faculty explain they engage students in thinking like a nurse. This approach has not proven to be useful for this purpose. In fact, there is insufficient evidence that the traditional approach to clinical education meets the needs of nursing students (Ironside, McNelis, & Elbright, 2014; Leighton, et al, 2021).

> During clinical, students should spend as much time thinking as performing tasks.
>
> Nurses think 100% of the time!
>
> How much time do we allow students to pause from performing tasks to engage in clinical judgment?
>
> The literature reveals students spend very little to no time thinking while in the clinical setting.

Although teaching clinical judgment has received a lot of attention in the nursing literature over the last 5 years, the teaching/learning strategies presented typically do not include any used in the clinical. As previously noted, Nielsen et al (2023) conducted a study to determine the current practices for teaching clinical judgment. That research revealed there are very few strategies described in the literature for teaching clinical judgment in clinical settings.

This is a real problem. When students graduate, they will be expected to think in the practice setting, yet they are not given opportunities to use clinical judgment in the clinical setting while in school.

Students must be guided in how to think during their clinical learning experiences! A perfect way to do this is to use "cognitive guidance" tools to help students apply clinical judgment competencies (thinking skills). The Appendices of this book includes an example of a cognitive guidance tool that applies the clinical judgment competency (thinking skill) of "judging how much ambiguity can be tolerated in a situation." This is one of 23 clinical judgment competencies in the Caputi Clinical Judgment Framework.

To further emphasize clinical judgment, faculty can adopt the concept map approach as previously discussed under the Principle: Replace 5-column care plans with concept maps.

Nurse educators must not be fearful of changing the "way we have always done it" to incorporate new, innovative ways for teaching nursing.

PRINCIPLE

#33 Memorization of factual information outside of a context can lead to inaccurate application of the information to real situations.

John Dewey was a pioneer in education in the United States. As faculty at the University of Chicago he contributed new ideas to established educational pedagogy. Dr. Dewey may have been the first to advance the idea expressed in this Principle—that learning factual information must be accomplished within a context for that factual information to be meaningful. This Principle has been reinforced and applied to nursing education by many writers across the last three decades, but most notably by Dr. Benner and her colleagues in the 2010 publication, *Educating Nurses: A Call for Radical Transformation*.

Nursing education has evolved over the years from sage on the stage (lecturing), to guide on the side (active involvement), to team on the screen (online learning). A major focus for classroom teaching today is to actively involve students during class time. This does not mean that faculty never lecture, but that faculty no longer spend hours lecturing and never actively involving students in using the information to solve patient care problems. We must position the nursing content we teach within a context to demonstrate the meaning of that content. Teaching contextually could involve a patient case study, a problem on the nursing unit, or a collaboration issue when working with another healthcare provider.

Teaching just nursing content has no meaning; students must understand how that content relates to nursing practice. They must experience **how** the nurse uses the information rather than just knowing the information. Giving an example by explaining a case study or sharing how faculty used that information in their own experience is helpful, but that is passive and not active. Students must actively use the information in the classroom before they are called upon to use that information in the clinical setting.

Remember that memorization of factual information outside of a context can lead to inaccurate application of those factors to real situations. This is another reason why classroom application of content to patient situations is so important. Contextual learning makes learning meaningful. Teach content within a context. Provide students practice using applying and higher cognitive level activities within a context by using active learning strategies in the classroom.

Teaching just nursing content
has no meaning;
students must understand
how that content relates
to nursing practice.

Contextual learning makes
learning meaningful.

PRINCIPLE

#34 For deep learning to occur, the student must be actively engaged.

Learning is an inside job!

One reason active learning has become popular is that students learn more when they are actively engaged. Active engagement requires students to cognitively engage to recall information and use that information, rather than passively listen to a teacher lecture for prolonged periods of time. Students become "passive" learners when listening to a lecture. They are active learners when engaging in classroom activities that require them to recall information, analyze data, and use clinical judgment to apply content and data to a patient care situation or to solve a non-patient related nursing issue. Requiring **students to actively retrieve** previous learning from memory has two profound benefits:

1. It tells students what they know and don't know; provides information about where to focus further study to improve weak areas.

2. Recalling what has been learned causes the brain to **reconsolidate** the memory which strengths its connection to what is already known and makes it easier to recall in the future.

Learning is an inside job; therefore, the more students do in the classroom and the more faculty require them to **actively** recall previously learned information then apply that information using active learning (rather than passively hearing the faculty present and review material), the more learning will actually occur. The idea of students **actively** retrieving information is critical for student learning. This alone can help students retain and recall information putting them in a better position to be successful.

> Students learn more when they are actively engaged.

A good source of information on retrieval theory is the book *Make it Stick* by Brown, Roediger, and McDaniel (2014). This book presents many ideas for planning ways to build on previous learning, add new information, and engage students in continuous review. Also review RetrievalPractice.org. Lots of good ideas.

PRINCIPLE
#35 Not all active learning activities are equal.

Engaging students in contextual learning is part of active learning in the classroom. When using active learning, it is important to involve students in activities that require applying and higher levels of thinking. The lower cognitive levels of remembering and understanding are helpful as "drill and practice" activities when your goal is for students to memorize content. Although helpful as a memorization technique, drill and practice activities do not mimic the type of thinking a nurse uses in practice. The majority of active learning activities should require students to use the content in the way nurses use the content in practice. Identifying the level of thinking required when engaging in an activity is key to planning and/or developing active learning strategies to be used in the classroom.

Important point:

Active learning strategies should engage students in **thinking at the applying and higher levels** so the **type** of active learning matters. Some faculty report they engage active learning by using various drill and practice games and other lower-level thinking activities. These are good for the goal of memorizing information, but not for encouraging higher level thinking. Just as you determine the cognitive level of test items when constructing an exam, you must do the same when engaging students in learning activities by identifying the level of thinking required to carry out that activity.

> Identifying the level of thinking required when engaging in an activity is key to planning and/or developing active learning strategies to be used in the classroom.

PRINCIPLE

#36 Repetition with rote memorization does not support long-term memory and recall at a later time.

This principle was adapted from the book *Make it Stick* which says: "Repetition by itself does not lead to good long-term memory" (Brown, Roediger, & McDaniel, 2014, p. 8).

When teaching psychomotor skills, faculty typically demonstrate the skill, ask students to practice the skill, provide students feedback on their practice, then ask students to continue practicing until their assigned time to "checkoff" the skill. A checkoff typically means the student memorizes dozens of steps to perform the skill, then demonstrates those memorized steps in the presence of an instructor. Once students pass their checkoff, months may pass before they perform the psychomotor skill in the clinical setting. When called upon to perform the skill, faculty often observe students do not remember what to do and do not perform well. The student is sent back to the skills lab to practice. This is often referred to as skill decay (Kardong-Edgren, Oermann, & Rizzolo, 2019). This situation demonstrates that gains achieved during massed practice are transitory and melt away quickly (Brown, Roediger, & McDaniel, 2014).

What can faculty do? Rather than repeated practice of the skill until the student tests on the skill, perhaps teach the skill, watch students practice that skill with faculty oversight rather than performing a checkoff. Faculty correct student performance. The student continues to practice until the faculty is satisfied with the performance. Students then take the skills sheets to clinical. Faculty ask students to review the skills sheet and determine how the performance of that skill might need to be modified should their assigned patient need that nursing procedure. Students address questions such as: (1) What steps should be modified for this patient? (2) How will you modify the steps for this patient? (3) What steps cannot be modified and why?

With this approach students are reviewing the cognitive aspect of the skill. Once each term students are required to practice the skills in the skills lab. This approach requires intermittent recall and application to a variety of patient situations which is more effective for long-term memory and recall at a later time than lots of repetition without any further recall and application.

See the Appendices of this book for an example worksheet, *The Skill Decay Activity*, that can be used in the clinical for cognitive recall about how to perform the skill of insertion of a urinary catheter.

> Intermittent recall and application of learning to a variety of patient situations is more effective for long-term memory and recall at a later time than lots of repetition without any further recall and application.

PRINCIPLE

#37 The more students actively retrieve information, the more they will remember.

Faculty often begin a classroom session with a brief review of previously learned information. For example, if the topic for the day is care of patients with problems with oxygenation, faculty may spend the first 30 minutes of class time reviewing the anatomy and physiology of the pulmonary system. This type of passive review is not very effective or helpful.

Consider a different approach that reinforces what was written earlier in this book about homework. For homework preparation, students must actively retrieve previously learned information. Students complete worksheets that require them to review and record information related to anatomy and physiology that will be used in class that day. Faculty do not start the class with a review of the pulmonary system. It is important to call on each student throughout the class to share what they wrote on their anatomy and physiology review worksheets.

Review and recall of previously learned information should be performed by the students engaging in the retrieval process themselves. Student engagement in the tasks of review and recall is more beneficial than faculty reviewing previously learned information. As mentioned with an earlier Principle, learning is an inside job.

> Student engagement in the
> tasks of review and recall
> is more beneficial than
> faculty reviewing previously
> learned information.

PRINCIPLE

#38 Use the seven principles for good practice in undergraduate education.

The seven principles for good practice in undergraduate education, the classic work of Chickering and Gamson (1987), is still relevant in today's higher education environment. The seven principles are:

1. Encourage contact between students and faculty.

2. Develop reciprocity and cooperation among students.

3. Encourage active learning.

4. Give prompt feedback.

5. Emphasize time on task.

6. Communicate high expectations.

7. Respect diverse talents and ways of learning.

Although these 7 principles may appear to be "common sense," faculty may not be aware of them or even know to use them in the classroom. These seven principles have also been revised for online teaching.

It is important for faculty to dig deeper into each of these principles of undergraduate education and use them in teaching/learning activities. For ideas about how to apply these seven principles in the nursing classroom, refer to this URL from the University of Tennessee, Chattanooga: https://www.utc.edu/academic-affairs/walker-center-for-teaching-and-learning/teaching-resources/pedagogical-strategies-and-techniques/seven-principles-for-good-teaching.

> Although these 7 principles may appear to be "common sense," faculty may not be aware of them or even know to use them in the classroom.

123

PRINCIPLE
#39 Appeal to the students' emotions to foster intrinsic motivation.

Motivation is a key factor in student success. Intrinsic motivators are internal factors that represent the students' internal feelings and beliefs. Students are motivated to learn because they care about what is being taught and want to learn about the content. They are internally driven. Contrast extrinsic motivation. Extrinsic motivation is driven by an external reward such as points for homework or grades on an exam or research paper. Motivators that result in long-lasting learning are those driven by intrinsic factors. Appealing to a student's emotions is a powerful stimulus for intrinsic motivation. Here is an example.

While teaching Fundamentals in Nursing, I became aware that most the students were excited to learn nursing and were motivated by the media's view of nursing—fast-paced, emergency and critical care nursing. They were often bored and unmotivated when learning about caring for elderly patients in a long-term care setting. I realized I had to appeal to their emotions. I was teaching at College of DuPage, an institution that was very supportive of faculty-produced learning materials. The college provided a photographer. The photographer and I visited a long-term care facility. With permission, the photographer took pictures of an elderly resident of the nursing home with her very caring nurse.

After the photo session, we assembled the pictures into a series of photos. The college hired a nurse (Deb Gauldin, www.DebGauldin.com) who is a singer and songwriter to write and perform the song "Tucked in Tight." We then put together a video of the pictures. The video displayed each picture in a planned order showing the caring nature of the nurse in her interactions with the elderly lady. As the video played, Deb Gauldin softly sang the song she wrote that talked about the care the nurse was providing the elderly resident. The lyrics of the song were directed to the patient's loved ones who were not with the elderly patient on a daily basis. The nurse sang, "Because you can't be here every day, for you I will tuck her in tight." At the end of the three-minute video there wasn't a dry eye in the classroom. The students were emotionally changed as was their attitude about caring for elderly patients in a long-term care setting. They learned in a very emotional way the value of nurses working in long-term care facilities and the value of the care they provided. Appeal to the student's emotions to foster intrinsic motivation.

Appealing to the students' emotions can shift attitudes.

Information about using the *Tucked in Tight* video to teach to the affective domain and to view the actual *Tucked in Tight* video is available at my website. You may play this video to students, **free of charge**, from my website: https://LindaCaputi.com and click on the Tucked in Tight tab. At that URL you can:

1. Project and play the video in your classroom so your students can witness the value of caring for the elderly.

2. Watch a video that explains the teaching/learning strategies used to appeal to the affective domain that meet the goal of internally motivating the students.

I sincerely hope you use the video and find it helpful in shifting students' attitudes when needed.

PRINCIPLE

#40 Putting it all together:
prior learning, current homework assignments, classroom lecture, and classroom activities.

Both student learning and student retention are strengthened with a consistent approach to classroom teaching and learning that builds and expands on previously learned information from the current course, prerequisite non-nursing courses, and prerequisite nursing courses. The era of teaching nursing courses in a "siloed" way is over. The era of students deliberately applying previously learned information has arrived. For example, when teaching a second semester course such as an adult health nursing course, require students to recall what they learned in the previous nursing courses from the first semester, but now apply that nursing content to adult nursing care. In subsequent terms compare how the foundational information that was applied to adult health nursing is used in the care of other patient populations such as pediatrics and mental health. This definitely supports why one course is a pre-requisite to the other, and engages students in **retrieval theory** which is very effective for bringing forward previously learned information.

As previously discussed, classroom activities should require students to use homework. Homework activities should be focused and deliberate. Students should process and make meaning out of textbook readings, videos, review of credible websites, and other homework activities. This is where "worksheets" are used. Worksheets focus students on the information that is most important to glean from the homework assignments. Students bring these worksheets to class for further processing. Of course, the amount of homework should be doable. For example, rather than assigning complete chapters, assign pages that are most important for students to read. There is always much information in a textbook chapter that does not need to be read.

I suggest using a scrambled classroom approach where students engage in "meaningful" homework. Then students apply the homework information during active learning in the classroom. Active learning and the flipped classroom are overused terms and faculty may be experiencing fatigue hearing about those approaches. However, the more students think, apply, analyze, evaluate, and create in the classroom, the more learning will actually occur. Students must **actively** recall previously learned information then apply that information using active learning rather than passively hearing faculty present and review material.

Active learning does not mean never using lecture. The **scrambled** approach to classroom teaching combines a limited amount of lecture with active learning activities. It is fine to intersperse short burst of lecture especially when:

1. There are areas of both content and application of content that are typically difficult for students to understand. Your prior experiences teaching the content can guide you on what those might be.

2. You are working through activities and it becomes evident that students are lost or not understanding. At that point you can pause and provide a brief lecture.

The value of active learning strategies lies in (1) the level of thinking (cognitive level) that students are required to use to complete the activity, and (2) students' use of homework preparation materials. Using a detailed clinical judgment framework that directs students' thinking while working through active learning activities is essential for preparing students to think—to become self-directed thinkers.

> The era of teaching nursing courses in a "siloed" way is over.
>
> The era of students deliberately applying previously learned information has arrived.

CHAPTER 5

Testing and Evaluation

IN MY EXPERIENCE, TESTING AND EVALUATION is the least favorite nurse educator responsibility. Life for both faculty and students would be more pleasant if measuring student achievement of learning outcomes would not be necessary. But it is, so we must deal with any angst this topic may bring.

A major source of stress for faculty is lack of confidence in writing test items. Confidence in writing test items has been diminished by a barrage of messages from various sources telling faculty they are not testing experts; faculty need others to take care of this task for them. The strength and frequency of this messaging has grown over the last 15 years. The longevity of this messaging means that faculty joining nursing programs have little or no experience developing assessment tools and have learned to rely on outside sources. Many faculty believe the messaging they hear and integrate the idea of not being a testing expert into their self-concept. This is not a good situation. Faculty can write great test items. They do not have to be an "expert" in testing and evaluation to carry out their responsibility of developing solid classroom exams.

A major goal of this chapter is to change that messaging. I have worked for decades with faculty who have learned to develop assessment tools including how to write excellent test items for classroom exams. Not only can faculty develop their skills and become good test item writers, it is their responsibility to do so. It is not the job of an outside vendor to evaluate students' knowledge of what they are learning in the nursing program curriculum. That is the role of the faculty. And, it's not as hard as faculty are led to believe. You can do it!

Chapter 5 Principles

The Principles in this chapter will help guide you in the very important task of evaluating student learning.

PRINCIPLE

#1 Evaluation in nursing education serves a number of purposes.

I once saw a cartoon of an elementary school student handing his graded assignment back to his teacher. The grade on the paper was clearly an F. The caption of the cartoon said, "Miss Smith, which of us really failed here?" This is a very interesting comment to consider.

All student evaluation methods in nursing education are used to gather assessment data to determine if a student is achieving course and program learning outcomes. However, faculty can also use evaluation results for program improvement. For example, as you examine the results of an exam administered to various cohorts, look for common areas of weak performance. When similar weak areas are identified across several cohorts, use that information for ongoing program improvement.

If students across a number of cohorts have difficulty on an exam, perhaps the issue is not the students, but rather the way faculty taught the material. Faculty should consider how the content, and thinking using that content, were taught. Faculty must consider the cognitive level of the test items and reflect on their teaching to determine if students were provided practice using that content at the cognitive level of the test item. If the test item is truly an analyze level item, were students engaged in analyzing activities in class prior to being asked to analyze patient information on the exam?

Or, perhaps difficulty on the exam is a curriculum issue. Are the content and thinking expectations placed in the wrong course? Perhaps students do not have the prerequisite knowledge needed to learn the content and that subject matter should be moved to a course later in the program.

Another possibility is the test item itself may have been confusing or poorly written. It is critical that faculty receive student feedback on test items to determine how the student read the question. Students often interpret questions quite differently than the way faculty intended when the questions were written. To gain insight and learn to write better questions, faculty must allow students to explain the way they read the question. This information must come from the students. Faculty can engage students in several ways to collect this information. Two of these are the use of the *Loma Linda Exam Analysis Tool* and the *Student Test Response Form*. Both of these tools are in the Appendices of this book. Guidelines for using the Loma Linda Exam Analysis Tool are included with the tool in the Appendices. You can also access this tool at: https://lindacaputi.com/teaching-tools/.

> If students across a number of cohorts have difficulty on an exam, perhaps the issue is not the students.
>
> Use exam results for ongoing program improvement.

Use your students' exam results not only to address student weaknesses, but use exam results for ongoing program improvement and to become a better item writer.

PRINCIPLE

#2   It is best to develop a program-wide approach to testing in a nursing program.

It is always best practice to have a program-wide approach for writing test items, collecting quantitative test item data (such as the P value and point biserial index), analyzing the quantitative test item results, and making decisions about item analysis data. The policy can also contain information about reviewing the exam with students and the process for student remediation. Example items to include in a program-wide policy include:

1. A test blueprint and how to complete it (see the *Example Test Blueprint* in the Appendices of this book).

2. Determining the cognitive level of a test item.

3. Aligning test items to course learning outcomes and lesson objectives.

4. Guidelines for test item construction including the types of item formats.

5. If a pre-licensed nursing program, ensuring all exams use NCLEX style questions throughout the program. Define and describe what is meant by "NCLEX style" questions so all faculty are writing test items in the same way.

6. A process for reviewing test items prior to administering to students.

7. The type of quantitative item analysis data to collect.

8. How to analyze the item analysis data.

9. Acceptable ranges for item analysis data.

10. Actions to take based on the item analysis data.

11. The approach to reviewing exams with students.

12. The process for remediating students based on their scores. For example, all students earning 80% or lower must meet with faculty to review the exam and complete the Exam Analysis Tool.

13. How to conduct teacher-mediated remediation.

14. Identifying areas of weak performance by the group and how to address those weak areas in subsequent classes as a form of group remediation.

15. Integrating the content of weak performance areas into subsequent lessons.

An example of some of the above, and more, presented in the form of a testing policy is included in the Appendices of this book—*Example Items for a Program-wide Testing Policy.* The example is not all inclusive. The intention is to provide examples of more specific information related to classroom exams than included in this Principle.

Develop a program-wide approach for writing test items, collecting quantitative test item data (such as the P value and point biserial index), analyzing the quantitative test item results, and making decisions about item analysis data.

A consistent approach leads to better outcomes.

As mentioned throughout this book, consistency is key to success in a nursing program. Students especially appreciate consistency in test item construction so they can focus on what the test items are asking, rather than adjusting to a different way of testing depending on the faculty writing and administering the exam. It is best when all faculty use the same approach to exam development, analysis, and remediation. Consistency is key for all aspects of a quality nursing program.

PRINCIPLE

#3 Become familiar with linguistic modification and linguistically modify your exam questions as needed.

Nursing faculty have a moral responsibility to develop fair exams with clearly stated items (Moore & Clark, 2016). This may be a challenge for faculty when writing exams. What may appear to be a clearly stated item to faculty may not be clearly stated to students. Students often label difficult to understand questions as "trick questions."

Faculty have lots of nursing experience and are able to quickly grasp what is being asked. This is not the case for students. Consider these two test item stems that appeared on a Practical Nursing exam I reviewed for a nursing program in my work as a nursing education consultant.

1. "In which situation should the nurse have a high index of suspicion for water intoxication?"

2. "Which of the following will a nurse teach to a patient with chronic obstructive pulmonary disease to empty the lungs of used air and promote inhalation of oxygen?"

Students found both these items confusing. Both items can benefit from linguistic modification.

A reliable nursing exam requires the items to be written so students understand what the item is asking. Students should not be challenged to interpret complex English language. The first item includes the phrase "a high index of suspicion," a phrase that may not be familiar to the pre-licensure nursing student. The second item is a long sentence that takes time to decipher. That one sentence can be divided into a sentence and a question for easier processing.

If students answer a test item incorrectly it should be because they do not know the content or cannot think at the required level. They should not answer incorrectly because they do not understand what the question is asking. Exams should test the student's knowledge and application of nursing—not mastery of complex language. The students' ability to process higher level English language can be assessed by other means such as reading a research article and discussing its implications. Exams are a stressful event. Using complex English language when writing the item affects the reliability of the item because students may answer incorrectly because they have difficulty interpreting what the question is asking rather than not knowing the content or able to think at the level required of the test item.

Learn about linguistic modification. You can start by reading the article on the reference list by Moore and Clark (2016).

A reliable nursing exam requires the items to be written so students understand what the item is asking.

Students should not be challenged to interpret complex English language.

PRINCIPLE

#4   Learn what Bloom's taxonomy is really about.

Dr. Bloom's taxonomy of the cognitive dimension has been used in education for decades. In 2001 the original taxonomy was replaced with the revised version. For testing purposes, it is commonly accepted that a test item categorized at the apply or higher level is considered a critical thinking (clinical judgment) test item.

What is sorely lacking in nursing education are specific guidelines that all faculty in a nursing program use to determine the cognitive level of a test item. Some faculty believe the cognitive level of a test item is determined by the verb used in the stem. Using a specific verb does not ensure the student actually engages in an expected level of thinking.

I attended a webinar that focused on how to write Next Generation NCLEX unfolding case study questions. The presenter commented that if a test item is part of a case study, then it is automatically an apply or higher-level question. This statement is not correct. Does the item format (unfolding case study) determine the cognitive level of the test item? The answer is no. The item type does not make the cognitive level.

So, what does determine cognitive level? The simple answer is the cognitive level is determined by the type of thinking required to answer the question. If the student is able to merely recall information to arrive at the answer, then the cognitive level of that test item is remember. If the student must sort through information to distinguish relevant from irrelevant information or rearrange and structure information in the test item to determine the meaning of the information, then the test item is likely an analyze level item. To determine the cognitive level of a test item, identify the type of thinking the test item requires the **student** to use to answer the question, then align that thinking with the thinking described by Bloom's taxonomy to determine the cognitive level.

It is helpful for faculty to develop a process for studying Bloom's taxonomy and using it to determine cognitive level of test items. The process yields the best results if it is part of a faculty item writing policy that all faculty use across the nursing program.

To determine the
cognitive level of a test item,
identify the type of thinking
the test item requires
the student to use
to answer the question,
then align that thinking
with the thinking described
by Bloom's taxonomy
to determine the
cognitive level.

PRINCIPLE

#5   Assessments should align with the cognitive level expected in the course as expressed in the course learning outcomes.

My consulting work has revealed a weak area in nursing education is a lack of knowledge about how to determine the cognitive level of a test item. It is incredibly important that a test item is accurately categorized according to cognitive level. Faculty must ensure that test items are written at the applying, analyzing, evaluating, and creating cognitive levels of Bloom's taxonomy. If items are not written at these levels, faculty cannot determine if students are thinking at the levels required for practice and for what will be measured on the NCLEX.

Not including higher cognitive level test items on exams can also inflate grades. Students pass courses with inflated grades but are not prepared for practice and often fail the NCLEX. Faculty have a responsibility for ensuring students are taught clinical judgment, are self-directed thinkers using a clinical judgment framework, and are able to think at the applying and higher cognitive levels. Nursing course exams must accurately assess students' ability to think at the higher cognitive levels.

So how do faculty determine the cognitive level of an exam item? The process is this:

1. As suggested in Principle #4, study Bloom's taxonomy (Anderson, et al, 2001).

2. Know the thinking required at each level of the taxonomy.

3. Determine the type of thinking required to answer the test item.

4. Determine which level of Bloom's taxonomy requires the same type of thinking as the test item requires.

5. Label that test item according to the matched cognitive level of Bloom's taxonomy.

For example, the remembering level of Bloom's taxonomy requires the learner to engage in thinking such as:

- Remember previously learned information.

- Recall factual information with no judgments.

- Merely restate memorized facts.

The applying level of Bloom's taxonomy requires the learner to engage in thinking such as:

- Apply concepts and theories as a basis for responding to the item.

- Remember and apply general ideas, rules, and theories.

- Interpret, demonstrate, or predict situations, processes, phenomena, and/or procedures.

The type of thinking required in all six cognitive levels must be determined, then faculty can align the thinking students must use to answer each test item to determine the cognitive level of the item.

Faculty must be able to determine the cognitive level of a test item and not take the labels provided by a testing company or a textbook test bank as the correct level.

Labeling of test items by these sources can be incorrect.

Faculty should make the determination about the cognitive level of a test item to ensure items are evaluating the students' ability to engage in higher-level thinking.

Please note, this same approach should be taken for determining the cognitive level required to complete learning activities in the classroom. As previously mentioned, classroom learning activities should be at the Applying and higher cognitive levels. Faculty must know the thinking required at each cognitive level to determine if the learning strategy engages students in the required thinking.

Assessment measures should align with the expected cognitive level of the students' thinking as expressed in the course learning outcomes.

PRINCIPLE

#6 To assist with the task of writing test items, compile a list of stems.

Writing good test items can be a daunting task. There are some activities faculty can do to help mitigate those feelings. One activity is to develop a list of stems. As I often say, nurses use the same approach to thinking for all types of patients. The difference is the patient information to which the thinking is applied. This is evident with the 2023 detailed NCLEX test plans. Clinical judgment is now an integrated process used across the entire test plan.

According to the NCSBN, integrated processes represent processes that are fundamental to all of nursing practice and everything the nurse does, so are integrated throughout the categories and subcategories of the entire test plans (NCSBN, 2023). Because clinical judgment is an integrated process, the 6 cognitive processes identified by the NCSBN that make up clinical judgment are the same for all patient care areas. This reinforces my mantra that "nurses use the same approach to thinking for all types of patients."

Clinical judgment questions should require students to think at the apply and higher cognitive levels. Putting a question in an "unfolding case study" format does **not** automatically make that question an apply or higher-level item. Each stem should be categorized according to Bloom's taxonomy as explained in Principle #5 in this chapter.

Each stem developed should also align with one of the NCSBN's cognitive processes of their Clinical Judgment Measurement Model. But remember, that model only provides 6 general thinking processes. Students must learn the detailed thinking of clinical judgment. Students must **first learn** the clinical judgment framework that teaches the detailed thinking, then faculty can expect students to answer clinical judgment types of questions. Just asking these questions without teaching the framework is unfair to students—you would be expecting them to apply thinking they did not learn.

Faculty can use the list of developed stems in all nursing courses. Stems also can be used more than once on an exam because each time the stem is used it will be covering different patient information. The thinking will be the same, but the content will be different. This is the same approach the NCLEX uses. Review the examples of the Next Gen format questions provided by the NCSBN. These same formats will be used many times over but with different patient situations.

Stems that relate to patient care and align to clinical judgment can be used across courses. As faculty develop a pool of test item stems, each stem should be categorized according to Bloom's cognitive level, step in the clinical judgment framework, and cognitive process of the NCSBN's Clinical Judgment Measurement Model. Faculty should provide an explanation about how the test item uses the thinking of the assigned cognitive level.

> Clinical judgment questions should require students to think at the apply and higher cognitive levels.

Here is the process:

1. Faculty write a patient scenario.

2. Once written, faculty use one of the example stems to construct the item.

The following table presents example stems aligned to the cognitive process of the NCSBN's Clinical Judgment Model, the step in the Caputi Clinical Judgment Framework, and the cognitive level according to Bloom's taxonomy.

Stem: First present a patient situation, then use one of the below stems.	Cognitive Process of the NCSBN Clinical Judgment Model	Step of the Caputi Clinical Judgment Framework and Specific Clinical Judgment Competencies	Cognitive Level According to Bloom
What further information will the nurse collect based on the patient's *(blood pressure; temperature; hemoglobin; new onset of confusion, etc.)*?	*Recognize Cues*	*Getting the Information* The specific clinical judgment competency is: Assessing systematically and comprehensively	*Analyze*
Which information in the nurses' notes is relevant to the care the nurse will provide today?	*Analyze Cues*	*Making Meaning of the Information* The specific clinical judgment competency is: Distinguishing relevant from irrelevant information	*Analyze*
Determine which potential nursing intervention(s) is (are) most important for the care of this patient. Select all that apply.	*Prioritize Hypotheses* and *Generate Solutions*	*Determining Actions to Take* The specific clinical judgment competencies are: Selecting interventions and Setting priorities	*Analyze*

The analyzing level of Bloom's taxonomy requires the student to use some of these thinking skills:
- Break down and analyze the information; uses two or more concepts to answer; set priorities.
- Discriminate complex information.
- Categorize the structure or organization of ideas; identify the relationship of these parts as a whole.
- Examine cause-and-effect relationships.
- Detect recurring themes.

These thinking skills are needed to process the test items based on what the stem is asking. That type of thinking aligns with the analyze level of Bloom's taxonomy.

This type of pre-established information is very helpful to faculty as they write test items. This table can be part of a "test stem" document. Faculty must write the patient scenario, the correct answer(s), and the distracters. However, a large part of the task of writing a test item is completed with established pre-written stems and cognitive level assigned.

Some of the content in the table is taken from the faculty resource materials that accompany the student textbook *Think Like a Nurse: The Caputi Method for Learning Clinical Judgment* (2022) used with permission.

PRINCIPLE

#7 Be accepting of the question, "Is this going to be on the test?"

A common annoyance for faculty is when students ask, "Is this going to be on the test?" As a new faculty, that question once annoyed me as well until I started reading about motivation theory. The test represents an extrinsic motivator as discussed in an earlier Principle in this book.

An extrinsic motivator in education is the external reward of earning a passing grade on an exam. Successful completion of all exams and courses serves to achieve a bigger reward—earning the degree and gaining employment as a licensed nurse. Extrinsic motivators matter to students so should matter to faculty as well. I soon learned to respect the students' question, "Is this going to be on the test?"

> Extrinsic motivators matter to students, so they should matter to faculty as well.

PRINCIPLE
#8   Focus more on assessment than on grading.

"Focus more on assessment than on grading. Assessment is **for learning**, not for determining if competencies were met or for calculating final course grades. Assessment for learning is formative—a process by which you provide feedback to students to improve their performance and promote their learning. Assessment is more important than evaluating the outcomes of learning and deriving grades (summative evaluation)." Dr. Marilyn Oermann, personal communication, October, 2022, used with permission.

Perhaps the assessments Dr. Oermann is referencing are not performed frequently enough to inform faculty about student learning. Using technology such as "clickers" to poll the class to determine degree of learning is one formative assessment technique that can be used. Also, engaging students in active learning in the classroom and post-simulation debriefing are also ways to gather assessment data to drive further teaching.

Of course, grades are a necessary part of education, so eventually summative evaluation must be used to collect assessment data and assign a grade. Exams are used throughout a course for this purpose.

I often times hear that faculty do not review course exams with students because:

1. They are worried about test integrity.

2. It takes too much class time.

3. Students do not want to make appointments during faculty office hours so there is no time to review course exams.

As Dr. Oermann points out, assessment is for learning. Students must have feedback on their exam performance and how they might improve. Misunderstood nursing content must be clarified, and inability to think at the level required by an exam item must be corrected. Additionally, students must analyze their test taking skills and develop a plan for improvement so their exam scores will improve.

You can make this happen. Consider using the Exam Analysis Tool developed by faculty at Loma Linda University. Refer to the Appendices for a copy of this tool or access that tool at: https://lindacaputi.com/teaching-tools/. Ingram, et al, (2022) found that using this exam analysis tool resulted a positive change in grades across the course to the final exam. Her study also indicated that retention increased to 90%.

Assessment is part of the teaching/learning process and is another means for faculty to help students learn.

> Students must have feedback on their exam performance and how they might improve.
>
> Misunderstood nursing content must be clarified, and inability to think at the level required by an exam item must be corrected.

PRINCIPLE

#9 Exams results should always be used to help students learn.

As mentioned in Principle #8 in this chapter, students must review their exams and engage in further learning about content they missed as well as deficiencies in thinking abilities based on the cognitive level of incorrectly answered test items. Exams are an important learning tool for students. Students must review their test results, identify areas of weakness in their content knowledge, identify how to improve their thinking, and learn to be better test takers.

Although it is helpful for students to read rationales for the correct and incorrect answers, that is not enough to really make an exam a learning tool. There are many aspects of a test item including:

- Knowing the content referenced in the test item

- Thinking at the level required to answer the question

- Understanding what the stem is asking

- Knowing all the terms and words in the stem and answer options

- Determining which options are correct and why

- Determining which options are incorrect and why

Just reading rationales for the correct and incorrect answers is **not** the end-all to test review. There are no guarantees students actually increase their knowledge and thinking levels by reading rationales.

1. Rationales are helpful only to the extent they explain what the faculty (or another item writer) was thinking when writing the item.

2. Rationales typically only focus on content and not on the level of thinking required.

3. Rationales do not necessarily correct or improve the students' weak areas related to either content or thinking.

4. Rationales do not clarify any misunderstandings students may have had about the way the question was worded or exactly what the question was asking.

Additionally, results of the exam should be used to address weak areas in performance by the group of students. When test results indicate the students as a group did not perform well on specific content, faculty should pull into the following weeks' discussions that weak content. **Addressing this weak performing content should not just be a review of that content as used on the exam, but further application of that content to other patient situations in the course.** This works to provide strengthening of these weak content areas for the group as a whole. The same approach should be taken for cognitive level of test items. If analysis of exam results indicates the students scored poorly on analysis level test items, in the several weeks following the exam and prior to the next exam, faculty should engage students in analysis level activities in the classroom. Using these interventions, faculty are using exam results for remediation not only for individual students, but for the group as a whole.

> Addressing weak performing content should not just be a review of that content as used on the exam, but further application of that content to other patient situations in the course.
>
> The same approach should be taken for cognitive level of test items.
>
> These weak areas of performance can also be revisited in subsequent courses.

The above process should be applied to all exams and also to the results of the final exam in a course. The final exam results should be analyzed for weak areas of performance of the cohort. Those weak areas (content and thinking) should be revisited in the next courses. It is important to revisit and reinforce any content and thinking gaps as the students move forward.

PRINCIPLE

#10   All assessment methods must be valid and reliable.

A **valid** assessment method is one that measures what it is students are to have learned in the course. That is, a valid exam should assess the student's understanding of what has been taught, and what was taught should align to the course learning outcomes. An exam is not fair if it tests content or requires thinking that was not taught. An example is testing what clinical judgment is or expecting students to use clinical judgment to answer a test item when the concept of clinical judgment itself was not taught (Hensel, 2022).

For classroom exams, **validity** can be demonstrated with the use of a test blueprint that aligns each item to a lesson objective and each lesson objective is linked to a course learning outcome. This demonstrates the item assesses students' knowledge and thinking required for the course.

Reliability for classroom exams is typically demonstrated with item analysis statistics such as the P value (percent of students correctly answering the item) and the point biserial index.

To be **reliable** the assessment method must consistently measure the performance of students; that is, the results are comparable over time and are comparable among different learners and among different faculty teaching the content.

It may seem desirable for all students to answer a question correctly. Faculty may be pleased when 100% of students answer a question correctly. However, the higher the P value, the higher the chances the test item is too easy and cannot determine which students actually know the content and can think at the required level, and those who cannot. P values above 80% start to become unreliable and cannot differentiate between students "who know" and those who do not. An exam must be able to differentiate between students who know the content and those who do not so faculty know which students need academic support. Contrary, items with a P value too low are too difficult. An item with a P value less than 30% is likely too difficult and even the higher scoring students are unable to answer the question correctly.

The point biserial index of the correct answer indicates if students who scored the highest on the exam answered the test item correctly and those who scored the lowest on the exam answered the question incorrectly. A test item is reliable if those who scored highest on the overall exam answered the question correctly and those who scored lowest on the overall exam answered the item incorrectly. If students who scored poorly on the overall exam answered an item correctly more frequently than those who scored highest on the overall exam, then that item may be flawed and is not a reliable indicator of student learning. The more items that are reliable on an exam, the greater the overall reliability of the exam.

Most faculty have item analysis data readily available through their testing software. However, as with all program data, faculty must use the data to determine if the exam is reliable. Faculty should determine an acceptable range for the P value and for the PBI for both the correct and incorrect answers. Faculty must determine what to do with an item should the results fall outside the acceptable ranges.

> All assessment methods must be valid and reliable to render them fair measures of the students' learning.

The Appendices presents some additional information about a test blueprint and item analysis statistics.

PRINCIPLE
#11 Define what you mean by "practice ready."

Perhaps one of the purposes of evaluation of your students is to determine if—at the end of the program—they are "practice ready." The term practice ready is used frequently in nursing and nursing education, but it is not well-defined in the literature. Additionally, a universal definition and use of the term has not been established.

The definition and conceptualization of practice ready varies among settings. For example, a **regulatory agency** such as the National Council of State Boards of Nursing may determine a graduate is ready for practice after successfully passing the NCLEX. The NCLEX measures minimal competency for safe practice as a nurse. The **practice setting** may determine a new graduate is practice ready when the new nurse is able to take on, with minimal assistance, a patient assignment similar to the other nurses on the unit. The **educational institution** may determine students are practice ready when they complete the nursing program plan of study and graduate from the institution.

Because nurse educators interact with a number of these entities, it is best not to use the term practice ready or, if used, clearly define how the term is being used and what the term means to the user. As noted, the definition of the term varies across types of entities. Whether or not a new graduate is considered practice ready by the agency hiring the new nurse may be influenced by the perspective of the workplace. Perhaps the student is practice ready as defined by the educational institution, but the workplace is not ready to support the new graduate with a robust orientation and mentoring program, which the educational institution believes should be provided.

This lack of a definition of practice ready may contribute to the perceived education-practice gap that has been in the nursing literature for decades, but also is not clearly defined. So, what does the term education-practice gap mean? What are those gaps nationally, but also locally? One gap that appears to be pervasive across areas and levels of nursing is the ability to make clinical nursing judgments (Billings, 2019). Processes for closing this clinical judgment gap have been provided throughout this book. Primarily, students must learn a detailed clinical judgment framework with specific clinical judgment competencies (thinking skills) then apply that framework throughout all educational environments including in the classroom, simulation debriefing, and clinical. The approach to using the clinical judgment framework in clinical to connect the student's clinical judgment to actual practice was explained in the Principle: "Replace 5-column care plans with concept maps." This is an excellent example of revising a curriculum to address an education-practice gap issue with a process that puts the student in the actual role of the nurse. This type of change is critical for safe patient care.

> Both the terms
> "practice ready" and
> the "education-practice gap"
> are not well-defined.
>
> Determine what those terms
> mean to your nursing program
> and share your definition
> with students and
> your practice partners.

APPENDICES

1. List of Dr. Caputi's Principles

2. Loma Linda Exam Analysis Tool

3. Textbook Evaluation Tool

4. Student Self-Checklist for NCLEX® Success

5. Caputi's "Judging How Much Ambiguity can be Tolerated in a Situation" Cognitive Guidance Tool

6. The Skill Decay Activity

7. Student Test Response Form

8. Example Test Blueprint

9. Example Items for a Program-wide Testing Policy

Permission to use the tools in the Appendices.

Faculty who own a copy of *Dr. Caputi's Principles for Nurse Educators: A Guide for Teaching Nursing* may use these tools at the school where they are currently teaching. Use is restricted to the faculty's current place of employment. Permission is **not** granted for any other use of the tools in the Appendices. To use the tools in any other way, contact Dr. Caputi for permission at Linda@LindaCaputi.com or LindaJCaputi@gmail.com.

List of Dr. Caputi's Principles

Chapter 1: Who You Are as a Nurse Educator

Principle #1: Enjoy the moment; enjoy your moments of success in your role as a nurse educator.

Principle #2: Use the language of a student-centered teacher.

Principle #3: When we stop caring about our students, it's time to leave.

Principle #4: Ensure that students will always think of you as someone who made them feel good.

Principle #5: Earning certification as a nurse educator is a mark of excellence.

Principle #6: Be curious and grow from your inexperience. Find an area of nursing education that interests you and become an expert.

Principle #7: Nurse educators are "real" nurses.

Principle #8: Keep your passion for nursing education alive; be flexible.

Principle #9: Teaching nursing is NOT a retirement job!

Principle #10: Growing by small steps can lead to success as a nurse educator.

Chapter 2: The Workplace

Principle #1: The culture of the workplace matters.

Principle #2: After writing an angry email, read it carefully; then delete it.

Principle #3: Stay calm in the workplace.

Principle #4: Teamwork and collaboration is a QSEN competency that applies to nursing education at all levels.

Principle #5: Orientation as a new faculty is important; know what you need to learn.

Principle #6: Eat lunch with the new "kid."

Chapter 3: Accepting Change

Principle #1: Love what you do, but not how you do it.

Principle #2: We cannot keep doing the same thing over and over and expect different results.

Principle #3: The most dangerous phrase in the nurse educator's language is, "We've always done it this way."

Principle #4: Consider new ways of doing.

Principle #5: How do you eat an elephant? One bite at a time!

Principle #6: The status quo should never be good enough—always seek to improve your own performance and the performance of your students.

Chapter 4: Teaching and Learning Practices

Principle #1: Develop an evidence-based, competency-based nursing curriculum.

Principle #2: It's all about consistency.

Principle #3: Know where what you are teaching fits into the overall curriculum.

Principle #4: Teaching too much content can interfere with student success.

Principle #5: Teach resilience – a term fairly new to nursing education.

Principle #6: The iGen students are not the first generation of students who do not read.

Principle #7: Ensure the reading level of the required textbooks is at or below the reading ability of your students.

Principle #8: Always make homework assignments doable and meaningful.

Principle #9: Guide students through their homework

Principle #10: Students should fail themselves; they should get no help from faculty.

Principle #11: Know your audience.

Principle #12: Identify pain points in your nursing program.

Principle #13: Nursing program admission criteria need to be fair and reliable.

Principle #14: New learning can only be based on what students have already learned.

Principle #15: Do you have a weed-out course?

Principle #16: Teach students that technology is important, but never more important than the patient.

Principle #17: Fewer than 10% of new graduates demonstrate entry-level competence for clinical judgment in practice (Kavanagh & Sharpnack, 2021).

Principle #18: Students should graduate from a pre-licensure nursing program as self-directed thinkers.

Principle #19: It's not the content that is tested, it's how the nurse uses the content.

Principle #20: Teaching clinical judgment is so important because it is used in all nursing situations.

Principle #21: Clinical judgment is the overarching concept in all nursing programs at all levels of nursing practice.

Principle #22: Replace 5-column care plans with concept maps.

Principle #23: Saying "It's just common sense" does not make sense to new learners.

Principle #24: We need not be afraid to question and reconsider.

Principle #25: All faculty in pre-licensure nursing programs are NCLEX coaches.

Principle #26: Provide an intense, in-house NCLEX preparation course focused on YOUR students' needs rather than use a canned, off-the-shelf review provided by an outside entity.

Principle #27: A high NCLEX pass rate is desirable but not at the cost of a good completion rate.

Principle #28: KISS—Keep It Simple Scholar!

Principle #29: Always know the WHY behind the WHAT.

Principle #30: Teach to current practice.

Principle #31: What happens in clinical stays in clinical.

Principle #32: Thinking must occur in the clinical setting with as much time dedicated to thinking as doing.

Principle #33: Memorization of factual information outside of a context can lead to inaccurate application of the information to real situations.

Principle #34: For deep learning to occur, the student must be actively engaged.

Principle #35: Not all active learning activities are equal.

Principle #36: Repetition with rote memorization does not support long-term memory and recall at a later time.

Principle #37: The more students actively retrieve information, the more they will remember.

Principle #38: Use the seven principles for good practice in undergraduate education.

Principle #39: Appeal to the students' emotions to foster intrinsic motivation.

Principle #40: Putting it all together: prior learning, current homework assignments, classroom lecture, and classroom activities.

Chapter 5: Testing and Evaluation

Principle #1: Evaluation in nursing education serves a number of purposes.

Principle #2: It is best to develop a program-wide approach to testing in a nursing program.

Principle #3: Become familiar with linguistic modification and linguistically modify your exam questions as needed.

Principle #4: Learn what Bloom's taxonomy is really about.

Principle #5: Assessments should align with the cognitive level expected in the course as expressed in the course learning outcomes.

Principle #6: To assist with the task of writing test items, compile a list of stems.

Principle #7: Be accepting of the question, "Is this going to be on the test?"

Principle #8: Focus more on assessment than on grading.

Principle #9: Exams results should always be used to help students learn.

Principle #10: All assessment methods must be valid and reliable.

Principle #11: Define what you mean by "practice ready."

Loma Linda Exam Analysis Tool

*Developed by faculty at Loma Linda University, Loma Linda, California. Used with permission.

The Exam Analysis Procedure

The following steps make up the exam analysis procedure:

1. The student and instructor/learning facilitator become aware that the student has a problem with taking exams.

2. The student requests an exam analysis (or you require it as a program policy).

3. The student and instructor/learning facilitator who is doing the analysis, discuss the LAP Summary of Exam techniques.

4. The student and instructor/learning facilitator go over each question which the student missed on the exam. The student uses the exam techniques to answer these questions. (The student does not look at his former answer or at the correct answer on the answer key).

5. The student and instructor/learning facilitator identify the main category and specific problem or contributing factor for why the student missed each question.

6. The instructor/learning facilitator records why each item was missed on the exam analysis worksheet.

7. The instructor/learning facilitator totals the number of items missed and the percentages for each specific problem and each main category.

8. Suggested interventions are developed with input from the student and recorded on the Suggestions to Improve Exam Performance checklist.

9. A copy of the exam analysis is given to the student, and another is retained in the student's record.

10. Follow-up appointments (or referrals) for help with exam skills, tutoring, counseling and evaluation of progress are made.

Summary of Exam Techniques for Multiple Choice Questions

A. Be Sure You Know What The Question is Asking
- Read question carefully.
- <u>Underline</u> important words.
- Try to answer the questions yourself <u>before</u> you look at the answer options.
- Create a pool of possible answers (jot down key word(s) for each)

B. Consider Each Option Carefully
- Compare answer options given on exam with your own pool of possible answers.
- Re-read the question carefully.
- Read the answer options carefully underlining key words.
- Mark each answer option as either true, false, T?, F?, or ?.

C. Use Your Knowledge When Choosing the Best Answer
- Choose your answer based on what you have learned in the course.
- Do not choose an answer just because "it sounds good" if you have not heard of it before (in lecture or textbook)—it may be a cleverly worded distractor.

D. Use Your Time Wisely
- Do not spend too long on any one question.
- Read the question and answer options carefully (twice if necessary).
- If you are not sure which choice is correct, guess and mark the question number so you can come back to it if you have time.
- Do not be in a hurry to leave. Check your paper to be sure you have answered all questions.
- Check carefully for clerical errors (marking wrong answer by mistake).
- Read each stem with the answer you have marked to be sure it makes sense.

E. If You Do Not Understand The Question or Answer Option Ask For Help
- Ask the instructor to clarify what is not clear.
- Ask the instructor to "restate" a confusing question or option.

F. Do Not Change Your Answers Unless there is Reason
- The only time you should change an answer is when you know <u>why</u> the first answer is wrong and/or <u>why</u> the second answer is right.
- Never change an answer just because you feel uncertain.

Objective Exam Analysis Worksheet

Student _____

Course _____ Exam _____

Grade _____ Date _____

Test item missed	Lack of Knowledge						English Skills				Exam Anxiety				Exam Skills								Other (specify)	Analysis Results
	Reading/textbook	Inadequate notes	Application of knowledge	Poor retention	Other		Reading comprehension	Reading speed	Vocabulary	Other ___	Decreased concentration	Mental block	Forgot to use exam techniques	Other ___	Did not focus on what question asked	Failed to consider options carefully As T, F, ?, T?, or F?,)	Poor use of time	Changed answer	Carelessness/clerical errors	Did not write own answer first	Other ___	Other ___	
**																								
Items																								
%																								
% Totals																								

**Include more rows as needed.

Suggestions to Improve Exam Performance _____

_____

_____

_____

_____

_____

Name:_____ Date: _____ Class:_____

Priority # _____ **Lack of Knowledge of Subject Matter**

_____ 1. Use study guide/objectives/specific class guidelines to identify important content while reading textbook.

_____ 2. Write out key points from #1 and use for later review.

_____ 3. Take careful notes during class.

_____ 4. As soon as possible <u>after class</u> and at <u>the end of each week</u> review #2 and #3 from above

_____ 5. Participate in study group each week.

_____ 6. Use NCLEX review books to review important content and to practice application on review questions.

_____ 7. Predict exam questions. Use these for group review.

_____ 8. Schedule time to review each lecture carefully before each exam.

_____ 9. Note weak areas such as pathophysiology, medication side effects, lab values, etc.

_____ 10. Other: _____

Priority # _____ **Exam-taking skills**

_____ 1. Read each question carefully and <u>underline or circle key words</u>.

_____ 2. Give your <u>own answer</u> (write down a few words BEFORE looking at choices given on exam).

_____ 3. Mark each answer choice as T, F, ?.

_____ 4. Choose the best answer based on what you learned in this class.

_____ 5. Don't change an answer unless you <u>know why</u> the first answer is wrong. (<u>Never</u> change an answer just because you <u>feel uncertain</u>).

_____ 6. <u>Practice application</u> of knowledge using <u>case studies and NCLEX review questions</u>.

_____ 7. Other: _____

Priority # _____ **English Language/Vocabulary**

_____ 1. Look up vocabulary terms/new words identified in reading assignment, lecture, and study groups, etc.

_____ 2. Write out the meanings of these words, note pronunciation and use them in a sentence, make flash cards or write them in a notebook.

_____ 3. Drill on these words several times each week.

_____ 4. If you don't understand an exam question or answer choice ask the instructor for clarification.

_____ 5. Other: _____

Priority #_____   Exam Anxiety

_____   1. <u>Over-prepare for exams</u> so that you feel <u>confident</u> about your knowledge.

_____   2. Use recommended exam skills on every question. This helps you think logically.

_____   3. Use positive self-talk- i.e. "I know these concepts", "I am going to do well on this exam".

_____   4. Don't spend too long on a difficult question. This lowers your confidence and increases anxiety. Read it carefully 2Xs, guess and move on to easier questions. Come back later if you have time.

_____   5. Remain calm, remember what you have learned and apply knowledge and exam skills.

_____   6. Practice relaxation techniques (deep breathing, etc.) so you can use them p.r.n.

_____   7. Other: _____

Priority #_____   Other (Please Specify Below):

Some of the issues that fall under the "Other" column include physiologic needs such as the need for rest, hydration, and food. Another commonly cited issue is difficulty with the math required for dosage calculations.

Condon, et al (2016) reported that students continue to cite faculty support as a perceived need. These authors recommend early intervention for students who need faculty support. This is a driving reason for using this tool with every exam so this need is identified early.

The faculty support recommended consists of psychological support such as caring, understanding, encouraging growth, being approachable, and demonstrating empathy. Faculty behaviors to provide this psychological support include being available to talk with students, clear communication, providing helpful feedback, using fair evaluation methods, helping students identify problems and resolutions, and serving as role models. Faculty support can **significantly** affect student success. All this support reflects a "student-centered" culture.

Textbook Evaluation Tool

Textbook Details

Name of course(s) in which textbook will be used _____

Name of textbook _____

Publisher and date of publication _____

Anticipated date of next edition _____

Cost of textbook without online resources _____

Cost of textbook with online resources _____

eBook available _____

Content

Current	yes _____ no _____
Accurate	yes _____ no _____
Consistent with program's philosophy and learning outcomes	yes _____ no _____
Learning objectives clearly stated	yes _____ no _____
Presence of chapter summaries	yes _____ no _____
Suggested learning activities	yes _____ no _____

Quality of learning activities (explain)_____

_____

_____

Clinical judgment activities   yes _____ no _____

If yes, describe. _____

_____

_____

End of Chapter Practice Items:

Do practice items have a label that indicates they are NCLEX-style items?

yes _____ no _____

Are practice items truly NCLEX-style as defined by the nursing program?

yes _____ no _____

Faculty resources available   yes _____ no _____

If yes, describe. _____

_____

_____

Organization, Presentation, and Clarity

Effective use of:

- Page layout   yes _____ no _____

- Tables, graphs, and charts   yes _____ no _____

- Index   yes _____ no _____

- Glossary   yes _____ no _____

- Appendices   yes _____ no _____

Support Materials

Online materials: yes _____ no _____

Quality of the online materials: _____

_____

_____

Case Studies: yes _____ no _____

Quality of case studies: _____

_____

_____

Test Bank: yes _____ no _____

Quality of test bank: _____

_____

_____

Test bank found on the internet: yes _____ no _____

   If yes, note URL(s): _____

_____

Question publisher about:

- How the test items are written.

- The process for determining the cognitive level of test items.

- Their efforts to keep these exams from being sold on the internet.

Language and Readability

Reading level:

- State in terms of grade level and source of information about reading level.

- If source is publisher, request information about how they determined reading level.

Internal analysis of reading level:

Appropriate for reading level of your students   yes _____ no _____

Appropriate print size   yes _____ no _____

Writing Style:

Logical   yes _____ no _____

Concise   yes _____ no _____

Fluid   yes _____ no _____

Student Review

It is extremely important to gather student reviews of the textbook because students are the ones who will use the book!

Ask students to rate the book on the following qualities:

1. Readability
   a. Is the book easy to read?

   b. Is the level of English language easy for you to process?

   c. Are you able to understand what you are reading?

2. Are the online resources helpful? In what way? If not, how are they not helpful?

3. Are the graphics, charts, and tables helpful?

4. Is this book better than the one currently being used?

It is helpful to have students review several books from different publishers to determine which books meet their needs.

Be sure to have students from all levels of academic abilities review the book. If students earning higher grades can read and understand the book, but students earning lower grades cannot, then the book is biased and should not be used.

Student Self Checklist for NCLEX Success: Completed Throughout the Nursing Program

NOTE: The success activities are examples.
You can change them as needed for your program.

Success Activity	Nursing 1	Nursing 2	Nursing 3	Nursing 4	Nursing 5	Nursing 6
Completed all "homework sheets." Saved sheets for review when studying for NCLEX.						
Earned 80% or higher on each exam.						
Answered Apply and higher questions correctly.						
Remediated areas of content with poor performance.						
Used exam analysis tool to identify ways to improve testing; developed a plan.						
Eliminated test anxiety.						
Used stress reduction techniques during exams.						
Eliminated negative self-talk before & during exams.						
Took responsibility for studying for each exam.						
Reached out to faculty to clarify areas of confusion prior to taking the exam.						
Developed a study schedule for classroom exams.						
Developed a study schedule for remediation after exams.						
If repeating a nursing course, arranged for a tutor.						
Completed case studies r/t content.						
Completed review r/t course content in NCLEX review books.						
Completed (insert number) NCLEX questions r/t course content.						
Able to apply the clinical judgment framework competencies to patient case studies and patients assigned in the clinical setting.						
Familiar with all pharmacology r/t content.						
Scored high on clinical judgment exercises in the clinical area.						
Practiced prioritizing/delegating r/t content in clinical area.						
Portfolio of test results and remediation completed.						
Others:						

Caputi's "Judging How Much Ambiguity Can be Tolerated in a Situation" Cognitive Guidance Tool

Gather the following information:

Age _____   Gender _____

CURRENT:

Blood pressure: _____

Pulse: _____

Temperature: _____

Respirations: _____

Pulse oximetry: _____

Last 24 hour of vital signs: _____

Normal vital signs for this patient: _____

Activity level: _____

Medical diagnosis: _____

Pre-existing conditions: _____

Medications *(complete the following for all medications this patient is currently taking)*:

    Name: _____

    Classification: _____

    Effect on any of the vital signs: _____

    _____

    _____

Procedures/treatments performed: _____

_____

_____

_____

Effect of procedures/treatments on any of the vital signs: _____

_____

_____

Pain level:_____

Process the information for discussion with your faculty
and to share in post-conference:

1. From the information you gathered, identify the most important factors that influence each of the patient's vital signs.

2. Are the patient's current vital signs acceptable? Explain.

3. Identify the low and high readings that would trigger intervention along with the correct rationale.

4. Determine interventions you would take in the event the patient's vital signs go outside of your low and high parameters.

Taken from Caputi, L. (2022). *Think Like a Nurse: The Caputi Method for Learning Clinical Judgment.*
Used with permission of author.

Grading Rubric for the Vital Signs Cognitive Guidance Tool

Performance Level	S	NI	U
Identifies the most important factors influencing each of the patient's vital signs.	Correctly identifies the most important factors influencing each of the patient's vital signs.	Explanation includes some but not all of the most important factors influencing each of the patient's vital signs.	Unable to identify the most important factors influencing each of the patient's vital signs.
Able to determine and explain if current vital signs readings are acceptable for the patient.	Correctly determines and explains if current vital signs readings are acceptable for the patient.	Explanation is close but not completely accurate about acceptable vital signs for the patient.	Unable to determine and/or explain if current vital signs readings are acceptable for the patient.
Identifies low and high readings that would trigger intervention along with correct rationale.	Correctly identifies low and high readings that would trigger intervention along with correct rationale.	Explanation is close but not completely accurate about high and low readings to trigger intervention; rationales somewhat correct.	Unable to identify low and high readings that would trigger intervention along with correct rationale.
Determines actions to take should the vital signs go outside the established parameters.	Correctly determines actions to take should the vital signs go outside the established parameters.	Explanation of actions to take should the vital signs go outside the established parameters is incomplete and/or inaccurate.	Unable to determine actions to take should the vital signs go outside the established parameters.

S = Satisfactory

NI = Needs Improvement

U = Unsatisfactory

The Skill Decay Activity~
Inserting an Indwelling Urinary Catheter:
Applying Clinical Judgment

Procedure Steps	Can the step be revised? Y/N If Yes, why is the revision needed?	How will you revise the step for THIS patient?
Pre-Procedure Steps		
1. Check the healthcare provider's order.		
2. Read the agency procedure.		
3. Gather equipment and supplies.		
4. Perform hand hygiene.		
5. Obtain assistance if needed.		
6. Identify patient according to agency policy.		
7. Explain the procedure to the patient.		
8. Provide privacy.		
9. Collect assessment data related to need for urinary catheterization.		
10. Gathers the necessary supplies: insertion kit, an extra pair of sterile gloves, blanket for draping the patient, light source, and an extra sterile catheter in the same size.		

Procedure Steps	Can the step be revised? Y/N If Yes, why is the revision needed?	How will you revise the step for THIS patient?
Steps in the Procedure		
1. Provide perineal care.		
2. Appropriately position patient.		
3. Open catheter kit and position catheterization tray appropriately.		
4. Set up sterile field, don sterile gloves, prepare sterile supplies, drape patient. Lubricate first several inches of the catheter.		
5. Clean the urinary meatus. Clearly visualize the urinary meatus.		
6. For a female patient, hold the labia open or for a male patient hold the penis at a 90° angle then insert the catheter into the urethra until urine starts to flow through the tubing. Insert another 1 to 2 inches.		
7. Inflate the balloon and ensure it is properly positioned.		
8. Secure catheter tubing to inner thigh.		
9. Safely hang drainage bag to the bed at a safe level to prevent backflow of urine.		
10. Observe the patient during the procedure for pain, discomfort, breathing problems, or any other issues.		

Procedure Steps	Can the step be revised? Y/N If Yes, why is the revision needed?	How will you revise the step for THIS patient?
Post-Procedure Steps		
1. Assess the patient's condition and response to the procedure.		
2. Ensure the patient is safe and comfortable.		
3. Perform hand hygiene.		
4. Talk with patient about the procedure and answer any questions the patient may have.		
5. Document the procedure and the outcome.		
6. Dispose of all supplies and trash.		

Discussing the Clinical Judgment Competencies Used

Listed below are some of the Clinical Judgment Competencies you may have used. Discuss how you used them. List any others you used and how you used them.

- Identifying signs and symptoms

- Assessing systematically and comprehensively

- Predicting potential complications

- Selecting interventions

Student Test Response Form

Date: _____

Course: _____

Item Number: _____

Do you believe the test item is clearly written or is confusing? Explain.

_____

_____

_____

Do you believe the answer key is incorrect? Explain

_____

_____

_____

Answer option you believe is the correct answer. Explain

_____

_____

_____

Documentation for information in your rationale such as textbook (page #), classroom notes (date), other course materials.

_____

_____

_____

Student Signature: _____

Example Test Blueprint

It is most important to align test questions to a **detailed objective on the NCLEX Test Plan and NOT just to one of the major 8 categories.

Question	Course Objective	Step in the Nursing Process	Detailed Objective on the Detailed NCLEX Test Plan**	Cognitive Level	Difficulty Level	Point Biserial Index (PBI) of the Correct Answer
1		Assessment		Apply	0.88	0.46
2		Diagnosis		Analyze	0.69	0.14
3		Intervention		Remember	0.73	-0.23
4		Diagnosis		Understand	0.88	-0.03
5		Diagnosis		Apply	0.91	0.42
6		Assessment		Analyze	0.94	0.19
7		Intervention		Analyze	0.5	-0.10
8		Intervention		Analyze	0.85	0.20
9		Diagnosis		Apply	0.91	0.11
10		Diagnosis		Remember	1.0	0.00
11		Evaluation		Apply	0.82	0.24
Etc.						

Add the information in the Difficulty Level column and the Point Biserial Index column on the blueprint after you administer the test and run the item analysis application. Use these statistics for improving your test items.

Summary:

Assessment	3	Remember	2	Difficulty Level		PBI 0.2 or higher	4
Diagnosis	5	Understand	1	Higher than 0.8	8	Less than 0.2	7
Planning	1	Apply	4	Less than 0.8	3	Positive	8
Intervention	3	Analyze	4			Negative	3
Evaluation	1						

The difficulty level is the percent of students that answered the item correctly. It is also called the P value. See Testing Policy for acceptable ranges.

Example Items for a Program-Wide Testing Policy

Overall Planning

1. Consider the overall curriculum and courses.

    a. Length of course.

    b. Amount of content in each course.

2. Determine the number of tests in each course.

3. Determine the number of items on each exam. Tests should be as long as possible to increase the reliability of the exam. Do not limit to a pre-determined number of items.

4. Each course will have a cumulative final exam.

5. Review the cognitive levels of the course learning outcomes and write questions at those cognitive levels.

Writing Test Items

1. A test blueprint will be used for all classroom tests. The blueprint will be completed while developing the test. The columns referring to item analysis will be completed after administration of the test. (See Appendix 8 of this book.)

2. All items will be written as NCLEX style questions. All NCLEX item types will be used.

3. Rationales for the key and distracters for all items will be written.

4. All items will be reviewed to eliminate test wise items.

5. All items will be reviewed using specific item writing guidelines.

6. All items will be linguistically modified as needed.

7. Items will be written as questions as much as possible. Completion items will be kept to a minimum.

8. Each option will begin with an upper case and end with a period.

9. The word patient will be used instead of client.

10. Items will refer to "The nurse" and "a patient".

11. Important words in the stem will be bolded or otherwise highlighted.

12. Only generic names of medications will be used.

13. All exams will be reviewed by another faculty prior to administering to students.

14. Faculty will consider the feedback and comments from the reviewing faculty to determine what changes need to be made.

Administering Tests

1. All student possessions (backpacks, cell phones, water bottles, hats, etc.) must be left at the front of the room.

2. Students are not permitted to sit at their desk with notes prior to the exam. Any last-minute studying must be conducted outside the classroom.

3. The teacher may bring an English dictionary for all students to use during a test. The dictionary will be accessed in the presence of the teacher. If knowing medical terminology is part of the question, the dictionary cannot be used for those words.

4. If a student is absent from a test, the student will take a different test than the one administered to the class. This test may be of a different format as well (essay, short-answer, etc.).

5. Simple, non-graphing, calculators without memory will be provided for dosage calculation items if not otherwise available.

Analyzing Test Results

1. The faculty who wrote the test is responsible for analyzing test results.

2. The following will be considered when reviewing item analysis data

    a. Item analysis

        i. P value (percent selecting the answer option): The acceptable range for the P value for the correct answer is between 50% and 80%.

        ii. All incorrect options (distractors) should have a P value to indicate some students chose the distractor. If no students chose a distractor, that distractor needs to be revised to make it more attractive to the uninformed student.

        iii. Point biserial index (PBI) guidelines

            1. The PBI for correct answers must always be positive.

            2. The following are ranges for the PBI of the correct answer

        a. 0.30 and above: excellent item

        b. 0.20-0.29: good item

        c. ≥ 0.19 is a poor item that needs to be reviewed and edited

     3. PBI for the incorrect answers should always be negative. If the PBI is not negative, the distractor needs to be revised.

   iv. Determine what actions will be taken if the stats are unacceptable

       1. Give credit for more than one choice. This is the preferred action.

       2. Nullify the test item by giving credit for all choices.

       3. Delete the test item from the exam and recalculate with one less total items.

    a. Exam KR-20: attempt to achieve 0.65 or higher.

3. These statistics will be used to determine the reliability of the exam. Items and exams without acceptable statistics will be reviewed and revised before using them in subsequent classes.

Reviewing Tests with Students

1. Test results will be returned to students no later than one week from the date of the test.

2. It is at the faculty's discretion if a group review is conducted. If so, the students will not be allowed to take any notes or take pictures.

3. Individual review

   a. All students earning less than 80% on an exam must make an appointment with the faculty for an individual review of the test.

   b. The faculty and student will use the Loma Linda Exam Analysis Tool (see Appendix 2) to determine what may have influenced the grade earned.

   c. The faculty will then discuss with the student the results obtained by using the Loma Linda Exam Analysis Tool to assist the student with strategies for improvement on the next exam.

   d. For each item missed, the student will use the textbook and class notes to write the rationale for each of the options.

   e. Faculty will work with students to individually remediate the content and thinking represented by the weak areas of performance.

   f. Students who do not follow this policy will be contacted by the faculty for a discussion of the importance of remediation for success in the nursing program.

Think Like a Nurse:
The Caputi Method for Learning Clinical Judgment

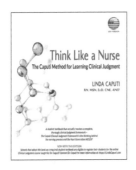 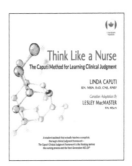

There are two versions of *Think Like a Nurse: The Caputi Method for Learning Clinical Judgment*. There is a USA version and a Canadian version. For more information please visit:

https://lindacaputi.com/about-the-book/

Research is now emerging that demonstrates use of the Caputi Method works to improve students' thinking. Here are a couple of reports.

- Dr. Huffstetler's (Brenau University in Georgia) dissertation reported that using the Caputi framework across a med/surg course after initially teaching the framework resulted in a statistically significant increase in the students' ability to engage in clinical judgment.

- Kaitlin Cobourne reports (in an article in progress) that making minimal curriculum revisions and incorporating the Caputi Clinical Judgment Framework in an associate degree nursing program resulted in NCLEX pass rates increasing from 68% to 92% in one year's time.

I invite you to learn more about the student textbook *Think Like a Nurse: The Caputi Method for Learning Clinical Judgment* by visiting my website at:

https://LindaCaputi.com and clicking on the clinical judgment tab.

You'll find information about the textbook and also about
the Caputi Online Clinical Judgment course.

Adams, M. (2015). Certification for nurse educators: A mark of excellence celebrating 10 years. *Nursing Education Perspectives, 36*(4), 207.

American Association of Colleges of Nursing (2021). *The essentials: Core competencies for professional nursing education.* AACN.

American Nurses Association. (2021). *Nursing scope and standards of practice.* Author.

Anderson, L. W., Krathwohl, D. R. Airasian, P W. Cruikshank, K. A., Mayer, R. E., Pintrich, P. R., Raths, J., & Wittrock, M. C. (2001). *A taxonomy for learning, teaching, and assessing: A revision of Bloom's taxonomy of educational objectives.* Addison Wesley Longman.

Benner, P., Sutphen, M., Leonard, V., & Day, L. (2010). *Educating Nurses: A Call for Radical Transformation.* Jossey-Bass.

Bernard, R. O., Rosales, M., & Zurcher, N. (2022). Exploring nursing students' motivation to prepare for class. *Nursing Education Perspectives, 43*(2), 118-120.

Billings, D. (2019). Closing the education-practice gap. *Health,* Wolters Kluwer retrieved January 2, 2023 from https://www.wolterskluwer.com/en/expert-insights/closing-the-educationpractice-gap.

Brown, P. C., Roediger, H. L., & McDaniel, M. A. (2014). *Make it stick.* Belknap Harvard.

Caputi, L. (2022). *Think like a nurse: The Caputi method for learning clinical judgment.* Windy City Publishers.

Chickering, A. W., & Gamson, Z. F. (1987). Seven principles for good practice in undergraduate education. *AAHE Bulletin,* p. 3-7.

Condon, V., Miller, E. M. W, Mamier, I., Zimmerman, G., & Ninan, B. L. (2016). Improving nursing students' academic performance through the exam analysis, In L. Caputi, (Ed.) *Innovations in nursing education,* p. 85-104. National League for Nursing.

Dickison, P., Haerling, K. A., & Lasater, K. (2020). NCSBN clinical judgment measure model clarification. *Journal of Nursing Education, 59*(7), 365.

Halstead, J. (2019), *NLN core competencies for nurse educators: A decade of influence,* Wolters Kluwer.

Hensel, D. (2022). Fair testing and incorporating next generation NCLEX items into course examination. *Nurse Educator, 47*(6), 352-353.

Ingram, D., Russell, K., Hill, K., & Daly, S. (2022). Enhancing exam performance to increase retention among students in an associate degree nursing program. *Nurse Educator, 47*(5), E105-E106.

Ironside, P., McNelis, A. M, & Elbright, P. (2014). Clinical education in nursing: Rethinking learning in practice settings. *Nursing Outlook, 62*(3), 185-191.

Kardong-Edgren, S., Oermann, M. H., Rizzolo, M. A. (2019). Emerging theories influencing the teaching of clinical nursing skills. *Journal of Continuing Education in Nursing, 50*(6):257–262.

Kavanagh, J. M., & Sharpnack, P. A. (2021). Crisis in competency: A defining moment in nursing education. *OJIN: The online journal of issues in nursing, 26*(1), Manuscript 2.

Kavanagh, J. M., & Szweda, C. (2017). A crisis in competency: The strategic and ethical imperative to assessing new graduate nurses' clinical reasoning. *Nursing Education Perspectives, 38*, (2), 57-62.

Leighton, K., Kardong-Edgren, S., & McNelis, A. (2021). Learning outcomes attributed to prelicensure clinical education in nursing. *Nurse Educator, 47*(1), 26-30.

Moore, B. S., & Clark, M. C. (2016). The role of linguistic modification in nursing education. *Journal of Nursing Education, 55*(6), 309-315. Doi: 10.3928/01484834-20160516-02.

Muntean, W. J. (2012). https://www.ncsbn.org/Nursing_Clinical_Decision_Making_A_Literature_Review.htm.

National Council of State Boards of Nursing. (2023). *Next generation NCLEX: NCLEX-RN test plan.* Author.

National League for Nursing. (2003). *Innovation in nursing education: A call for reform.* Retrieved from www.nln. org/newsroom/nln-position-documents/archived-position-statements.

National League for Nursing. (2012). *Outcomes and competencies for graduates of practical/vocational, diploma, associate degree, baccalaureate, master's, practice doctorate, and research doctorate programs in nursing.* New York: Author.

Nielsen, A., Gonzalez, L., Jessee, M. A., Monagle, J., Dickison, P., & Lasater, K, (2023). Current practices for teaching clinical judgment: Results form a national survey. *Nurse Educator, 48*(1), 7-12/.

Poledna, M., Gomez-Morales, A., & Hager, D. (2022). Nursing students' cue recognition in educational simulation. *Nurse Educator, 47*(5), 283-287.

Sieg, D. (2020). *7 habits of highly resilient nurses,* Sigma Theta Tau Nursing Center, https://nursingcentered. sigmanursing.org/features/more-features/Vol41_1_7-habits-of-highly-resilient-nurses.

Tanner, C. (2006). Thinking like a nurse: A research-based model of clinical judgment in nursing. *Journal of Nursing Education, 45*(6), 204-211.

Toffler, A. (1990). *Powershift: Knowledge, wealth, and violence at the edge of the 21st century.* Bantam Books.

Tyo, M.B., & McCurry, M. K. (2019). An integrative review of clinical reasoning teaching strategies and outcome evaluation in nursing education. *Nursing Education Perspectives, 40*(1), 11-17.

Uldrich, J. (2011). *Higher unlearning: 39 post-requisite principles for achieving a successful future.* Beaver's Pond Press.

Whittman-Price, R. A., & Gittings, K. K. (2021). *Fast facts about competency-based education in nursing: How to teach competency mastery.* Springer.

Made in United States
Troutdale, OR
06/13/2023

10589720R00111